Post-traumatic Epilepsy

Post-traumatic Epilepsy

Edited by

Marco Mula
St George's University Hospital and St George's University of London

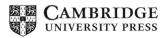

CAMBRIDGE
UNIVERSITY PRESS

CAMBRIDGE
UNIVERSITY PRESS

University Printing House, Cambridge CB2 8BS, United Kingdom

One Liberty Plaza, 20th Floor, New York, NY 10006, USA

477 Williamstown Road, Port Melbourne, VIC 3207, Australia

314–321, 3rd Floor, Plot 3, Splendor Forum, Jasola District Centre,
New Delhi – 110025, India

103 Penang Road, #05–06/07, Visioncrest Commercial, Singapore 238467

Cambridge University Press is part of the University of Cambridge.

It furthers the University's mission by disseminating knowledge in the pursuit of
education, learning, and research at the highest international levels of excellence.

www.cambridge.org
Information on this title: www.cambridge.org/9781108494229
DOI: 10.1017/9781108644594

First published 2021

Printed in the United Kingdom by TJ Books Limited, Padstow Cornwall

A catalogue record for this publication is available from the British Library.

Library of Congress Cataloging-in-Publication Data
Names: Mula, Marco, editor.
Title: Post-traumatic epilepsy / edited by Marco Mula.
Description: Cambridge ; New York, NY : Cambridge University Press, 2020. | Includes bibliographical
references and index.
Identifiers: LCCN 2020051500 (print) | LCCN 2020051501 (ebook) | ISBN 9781108494229 (hardback) |
ISBN 9781108644594 (ebook)
Subjects: MESH: Epilepsy, Post-Traumatic – etiology | Epilepsy, Post-Traumatic – therapy | Brain Injuries,
Traumatic – complications
Classification: LCC RC372.5 (print) | LCC RC372.5 (ebook) | NLM WL 385 | DDC 616.85/3–dc23
LC record available at https://lccn.loc.gov/2020051500
LC ebook record available at https://lccn.loc.gov/2020051501

ISBN 978-1-108-49422-9 Hardback

Contents

Contributors

Niruj Agrawal, MBBS, MD, MSc, FRCPsych
Department of Neuropsychiatry, St George's Hospital, London, UK Institute of Molecular & Clinical Sciences Research Institute, St George's University of London

Vincenzo Belcastro, MD, PhD
Neurology Unit, Maggiore Hospital, ASST -Lodi, Italy

Christopher M. Bonfield, MD
Vanderbilt University School of Medicine, Nashville, TN, USA
Vanderbilt University Medical Center, Nashville, TN, USA

Francesco Brigo, MD
Department of Neurology Franz Tappeiner Hospital, Merano-Meran, Italy

David K. Chen, MD, MPH
Baylor College of Medicine, Houston, TX, USA
Houston Epilepsy Center of Excellence, Houston, TX, USA

Hannah Cock, MBBS, BSc, MD, FRCP, FEAN
Institute of Medical and Biomedical Education, St George's, University of London, UK
Atkinson Morley Regional Epilepsy Network, St George's University Hospitals NHS Foundation Trust, UK

Cristina Rosado Coelho, MD, MSc
Setúbal Hospital Centre and Coimbra University Hospital, Coimbra, Portugal

Aristea S. Galanopoulou, MD PhD
Albert Einstein College of Medicine, Bronx, New York, USA
Montefiore Medical Center, Bronx, New York, USA

Derek D. George, MS
Vanderbilt University School of Medicine, Nashville, TN, USA
University of Colorado School of Medicine, Aurora, CO, USA

Colette Griffin, MBBS FRCP MD
Atkinson Morley Regional Neuroscience Centre, St George's University Hospitals NHS Foundation Trust, UK

Sarah E. Hall, BPsySc, MPsych, PhD
University of Melbourne, Victoria, Australia
Austin Health, Victoria, Australia

Peter Jenkins, MA, BMBCh, PhD
Epsom and St Helier University Hospitals NHS Trust, UK
St George's University Hospitals NHS Foundation Trust, UK
Imperial College London, UK

Anna Maria Katsarou, MD
Albert Einstein College of Medicine, Bronx, New York, USA

W. Curt LaFrance Jr, MD, MPH
Brown University, Providence, RI, USA
Rhode Island Hospital, Providence, RI, USA
Providence VA Medical Center, Providence, RI, USA

Simona Lattanzi, MD, PhD
Marche Polytechnic University, Ancona, Italy

Kimford Meador, MD, FAAN, FAES, FRCPE
Stanford University, CA, USA
Stanford Comprehensive Epilepsy Center, Palo Alto, CA, USA

Mariana Molero
Albert Einstein College of Medicine, Bronx, New York, USA

Marco Mula, MD PhD FRCP FEAN
Institute of Medical and Biomedical Education, St George's University of London, UK
Atkinson Morley Regional Neuroscience Centre, St George's University Hospitals NHS Foundation Trust, London UK

Jun Park, MD
University Hospital Cleveland Medical Center, Cleveland, OH, USA
Rainbow Babies and Children's Hospital, Cleveland, OH, USA

Michael Puntis, MB, BChir, MA, FFICM
St George's University Hospitals NHS Foundation Trust, London, UK

Genevieve Rayner, BA, MPsych, PhD
University of Melbourne, Victoria, Australia

Alfred Health, Victoria, Australia
Austin Health, Victoria, Australia

Patricia G. Saletti, PhD
Albert Einstein College of Medicine, Bronx, New York, USA

Zahra Sadat-Hossieny, MD
Stanford University, CA, USA

Alan R. Tang, BA
Vanderbilt University School of Medicine, Nashville, TN, USA

Jeevagan Vijayabala, MBBS, MD
Teaching Hospital Jaffna, SriLanka

Ximena Watson, BSc, MBChB, FRCA, FFICM
St George's University Hospitals NHS Foundation Trust, London, UK

Sarah J. Wilson, BSc, PhD, FAHMS, FASSA
University of Melbourne, Victoria, Australia
Austin Health, Victoria, Australia

Aaron M. Yengo-Kahn, MD
Vanderbilt University School of Medicine, Nashville, TN, USA
Vanderbilt University Medical Center, Nashville, TN, USA

Foreword

Epilepsy is a condition where individuals are prone to recurrent epileptic seizures. Of course, an epileptic seizure may be seen as a symptom, for which there are many different causes. We should therefore more accurately refer to the 'epilepsies' as a group of diseases. Head injury is a major cause of acquired epilepsy worldwide, particularly in resource-poor settings. Whether addressing prevention of head trauma, acute management, risk factors or the latent period prior to the development of the epilepsy, there are many areas where intervention could have an impact on overall outcomes.

This book brings together current evidence from a basic science as well as a clinical perspective with regard to head trauma and the development of post-traumatic epilepsy, collecting current evidence and addressing where it may sit with regard to management. As highlighted, severity of brain injury is a key factor in the likelihood of developing epilepsy, with an up-to 17-fold increased risk in those suffering a severe closed head injury and around a 50% risk associated with a penetrating injury. Despite this, relatively little attention has been given to this area, and it continues to be associated with poor psychosocial outcomes and high mortality. The book covers experience from animal models highlighting the different forms of head injury, translation to clinical care, and the multidisciplinary approach to address the prevention and management of morbidity and later onset epilepsy. It is timely in the light of ongoing international efforts to address risk factors as well as the unmet need.

This is one area where prevention of epilepsy is a real possibility; not only through the prevention and appropriate acute management of head injury, but also through recognition and intervention with regard to risk factors for the later development of epilepsy through biomarker recognition. What this book highlights is that the approach to post traumatic epilepsy is multifaceted; a collaborative approach is required to make an impact in future to reduce the prevalence and the associated comorbidities, so improving outcomes.

Professor Mula and the authors should be commended for this comprehensive piece of work.

Professor J Helen Cross MB ChB PhD FRCP FRCPCH OBE
Head, Developmental Neurosciences, UCL Great Ormond Street Institute of Child Health
London, UK
May, 2021

Preface

Epilepsy is one of most frequent neurological disorders, affecting about 50 million people worldwide, and post-traumatic epilepsy accounts for 10% to 20% of symptomatic epilepsies; nonetheless, research and clinical interest in post-traumatic epilepsy are still limited.

In order to find a volume with a similar title to this one, the reader would need to go back to 1949 with the publication of *Post-traumatic Epilepsy,* authored by Arthur Earl Walker, neurosurgeon, neuroscientist and epileptologist, remembered for the Dandy–Walker syndrome.

A PubMed/Medline search up to July 2020 using the search terms 'traumatic brain injury' AND 'epilepsy' generated 1,579 records against 3,032 for the combination 'traumatic brain injury' AND 'depression' and 6,458 for the combination 'epilepsy' AND 'depression'. It is therefore evident that attention to this topic is unsatisfactory despite not only the epidemiology of post-traumatic epilepsy but also the complex needs of people affected by this condition.

Research into this area has been rejuvenated during the last 10 years, especially regarding the management of traumatic brain injury, but this has only marginally improved the management of those who develop post-traumatic epilepsy.

Post-traumatic epilepsy is a complex condition requiring a multidisciplinary approach. Neurologists, neuropsychiatrists, neuropsychologists and specialists in rehabilitation medicine need to start working together and develop multidisciplinary coordinated clinical pathways to improve the care of people with post-traumatic epilepsy. This book intends to reflect these complexities, and for this reason it has brought together basic neuroscientists, neurologists, neurointensivists, neuropsychiatrists, neuropsychologists and specialists in rehabilitation medicine with either an epilepsy background or a traumatic brain injury background.

Chapter 1 is an overview of the basic neurobiological mechanisms behind the development of epilepsy after a brain injury. Chapter 2 reviews the epidemiology of post-traumatic epilepsy as well as current terminology in the light of the new International League Against Epilepsy (ILAE) definition of epilepsy and the difference between acute symptomatic seizures and late onset seizures. Chapters 3 and 4 cover the acute management of traumatic brain injury while the subsequent three chapters cover specific scenarios and subpopulations: post-traumatic epilepsy in children (Chapter 5), concussive convulsions during sport (Chapter 6) and traumatic brain injury during seizures (Chapter 7).

The subsequent four chapters are dedicated to the long-term cognitive and neuropsychiatric complications of traumatic brain injury and their potential role in post-traumatic epilepsy. Chapter 8 focuses on cognitive sequelae and rehabilitation strategies, and Chapter 9 on neuropsychiatric complications, while Chapter 10 discusses the relationship between traumatic brain injury and psychogenic non-epileptic seizures, a complex differential diagnosis and often coexisting problem in people with post-traumatic epilepsy. Chapter 11 focuses on the relationship between post-traumatic epilepsy and post-traumatic stress disorder.

Chapters 12 and 13 cover major problems connected to the pharmacological treatment of post-traumatic epilepsy: on the one hand seizure control and prevention, if possible, during the acute phase (Chapter 12); on the other hand, the effect of antiseizure medications on cognitive functioning (Chapter 13).

Finally, Chapter 14 focuses on major problems in managing post-traumatic epilepsy in low income countries. Around 85% of the world's population lives in medium to low income countries, and this has always to be in our minds.

The aim of this book is to provide a starting point for clinicians and researchers to discover again this syndrome. I am grateful to my colleagues who have enthusiastically joined this project, for sharing their expertise. I hope that this book will contribute to providing better care to our patients as well as improving the quality of life of their families.

Marco Mula MD PhD FRCP FEAN
St George's University Hospital
London, UK
July 2020

Chapter

1

Neurobiological Aspects of Post-traumatic Epilepsy: Lessons from Animal Models

Patricia G. Saletti, Anna Maria Katsarou, Mariana Molero and Aristea S. Galanopoulou

Introduction

Traumatic brain injury (TBI) is a common cause of emergency room visits for both adults and the pediatric populations, accounting for almost 2.5 million visits in the United States, a third of which are children.[1] TBI causes diverse brain pathological changes, whether direct or secondary to the initial injury, which include cell death, axonal and mitochondrial injury, inflammation, gliosis, neurodegeneration and synaptic reorganization that have been associated with epileptogenesis.[2–6] Seizures may occur immediately after the TBI (immediate or acute seizures) or during the first post-TBI week (early seizures). However, it is the occurrence of late spontaneous seizures, appearing after the first post-TBI week that establishes the diagnosis of PTE.[7–10] Post-traumatic epilepsy (PTE) may develop in 2–50% of patients that experience TBI. The rate of PTE increases with severity of TBI and with longer observation periods.[11, 12] Skull fracture, parenchymal brain lesions and intracranial hemorrhage, long period of post-TBI loss of consciousness, prolonged amnesia, age at TBI and – in several studies – acute post-TBI seizures have been linked with the development of PTE.[13–16] In addition to PTE, TBI can be associated with cognitive, neurologic or psychiatric comorbidities, like depression or anxiety that also greatly impact the quality of life and medical care needs.[17–23] PTE affects the patient's quality of life due to epileptic seizures, deficits in memory and cognition,[24–26] sleep disorders,[27] post-traumatic stress disorder, depression, anxiety and social behavioral changes.[28, 29] PTE is a devastating disease that still today remains without prevention or cure.[6] The latent period for the development of epilepsy following TBI seems to be important as a time window for prophylaxis pharmacotherapies to prevent the development of epilepsy.[6, 30, 31] The validation of methods that identify the time window for treatment and efficacy of drug effects is essential to translate to clinical trials. In this regard, studies with animal models are critical to elucidate the underlying mechanisms and pharmacological targets for therapeutic interventions in controlled experiments prior to clinical trial with epilepsy patients.

Here, we will review different animal models for TBI, with special emphasis on those that describe PTE development in rodents, highlighting the importance of each of them in the biological aspects post-trauma, comprehension of PTE development and preclinical trials for pharmacotherapies that may prevent and/or cure epilepsy following TBI.

A Comparison of Developmental Stages in Rodents and Humans

Rodents have a significant shorter life span, accelerated maturation and live in a different social environment than humans. The duration of gestation in rodents lasts 23 days opposed to 40 weeks in humans; eye opening occurs in postnatal days 13–15 (P13–15) rodents yet human newborns already have their eyes open; rodents start ambulating at 2 weeks whereas humans are able to do so at around 1 year of life; weaning from the dam in rodents takes place at P21 when breastfeeding in humans is usually during the first 6 months; life expectancy for rodents is up to 2 years whereas humans in the USA live approximately 80 years.[32, 33] Comparisons of brain developmental stages in rodents and humans has produced different results, depending on the criteria used to stage these processes. Using the maturation of the hypothalamic–pituitary–gonadal axis as a criterion,[32, 33] P0–6 are thought to correspond to the neonatal stage in rodents and P7–21 to infancy. Puberty begins around P32–36 in females and P35–45 in males, while adulthood is thought to begin after P60.[34, 35] The observation that around P8–10 the rate of growth of the brain and its DNA, cholesterol and water contents in rodents resembles that of newborn human babies had led to considering the P-10 rodents as equivalent to human newborn babies.[36, 37] However, discrete processes (timing of neurogenesis, synaptogenesis, gliogenesis, oligodendrocyte maturation, age-dependent behaviors, molecular and biochemical changes) mature with asynchronous trajectories within the brain across species challenging the concept that a single across-species staging method could apply for all developmental processes.[32, 33, 38–41]

Rodent Models of PTE

Fluid Percussion Injury

In the fluid percussion injury (FPI) model, a craniotomy is created at a specific skull region and when the animal starts recovering from anesthesia, it is connected to the fluid percussion device where a controlled pressure fluid pulse is delivered through the craniotomy, over an intact dura to generate TBI. Optimization and standardization of the conditions (anesthesia, size and location of craniotomy, pulse pressure) aim to simulate TBI of various severity levels and target specific brain regions. Acute mortality and acute post-TBI responses (apnea duration, first pain response, righting reflex), neurological exam outcome and acute post-TBI seizures are often used to describe the model characteristics. The FPI model reproduces several aspects observed in patients that suffered closed-head TBI with focal-diffuse injury.[17, 42] Table 1.1 summarizes some of those findings in animal models.

Studies that have utilized the FPI model for young rodents at different ages (PN17 and PN28) reported that the youngest animals appeared to have longer apnea period, higher mortality rate and hemodynamic changes than adult rodents.[41, 43] At older ages, the FPI is characterized by substantial structural damage to the impacted cortex (left parietal or right frontoparietal) and subcortical structures.[6] The FPI model has also been applied to neonate (PN1–5) and juvenile (3–4 weeks old) pigs for the investigation of the different cerebral hemodynamic responses after TBI.[41, 44]

Several behavioral comorbidities are observed in FPI model that are similar to what is experienced in TBI patients (Table 1.2). In both rats and mice of both sexes, FPI results in cognitive deficits,[18, 19, 21, 45–52] sensorimotor deficits,[18, 50, 53–55] sleep abnormalities,[56] anxiety[18, 21, 50, 52, 53, 57] or depressive symptomatology.[18, 19, 50, 57]

Cellular and molecular post-FPI changes that have been investigated for their role in epileptogenesis include alterations in the immune system, such as increased cytokine

Table 1.1 Rodent models of PTE

Model	Sex, species, age	Induction method (anesthesia, method)	Gross pathology	Acute post-TBI seizure-like events and mortality	PTE rate and characteristics	References
Fluid percussion injury models: lateral (LFPI), rostral parasagittal (rpFPI), central (cFPI)						
cFPI	Male – SDR, adult	Day 1: Pentobarbital, midline 4.8 mm. Day 2: Methoxyflurane, FPI 2.1–3.8 atm	- hemorrhages in corpus callosum, fibria hippocampi and thalamus; scattered petechial hemorrhages in brainstem	- acute mortality increases with pressure (10–100%) - acute seizure rate higher in nonsurvivors - EEG: after discharge of spikes 40–60 sec after FPI and suppression for 10–60 min post-FPI	ND	144
LFPI	Male – Harlan SDR, adult	Pentobarbital, LFPI 4 mm, severe (2.6–3.3 atm)		30% of rats have acute post-TBI seizure-like events	- PTE rate is 25% at 6 months; 50% at 12 months post-TBI - Mean seizure frequency was 0.3 ±0.2 seizures / day - 53–78% of PTE seizures are secondarily generalized	59, 63
LFPI	Male – LE Hooded rats, adult	Isoflurane, LFPI 5 mm,	- MRI changes in cortex, hippocampus,		- 30% of rats given severe LFPI developed	21, 51

Table 1.1 (cont.)

Model	Sex, species, age	Induction method (anesthesia, method)	Gross pathology	Acute post-TBI seizure-like events and mortality	PTE rate and characteristics	References
		moderate, severe, (3.2–3.5 atm)	thalamus, amygdala in LFPI rats - Large deformation high dimensional mapping of hippocampal morphometry differentiates PTE rats (lateral hippocampal region increase) from non-PTE (ventral and medial hippocampal decrease) - FDG-PET changes in ipsilateral hippocampus, 1 week to 3 months, may predict PTE rats		spontaneous seizures at 6 months post-LFPI - 52% of rats had epileptic EEG (SRS and epileptic discharges) at 6 months post-LFPI - Average of 6.3 seizures / 2 weeks - Mean seizure duration of 52.9 sec	
LFPI	Male – C57BL/6 mice, adult	Day 1: Pentobarbital, lateral parietal craniotomy 3 mm Day 2: Isoflurane, LFPI 2.9 ± 1.1 atm	- Cortical and hippocampal injury - Hippocampal injury in 56% of LFPI mice - No difference in Timm staining between controls and LFPI animals	- 10% acute mortality	**At 6 months post-TBI** - Up to 70% have epileptiform spikes - 58% have epileptiform discharges (rhythmic transients 1–5 sec)	53

| rpFPI | Male – SDR, P33–35 | Halothane, rpFPI 3 mm, 3.25–3.5 atm | 11% acute mortality

- Animals with focal GFAP staining under electrodes were excluded | with spikes and sharps).
- 3.2% (1/31) had SRS by 7 months post-LFPI

PTZ test, 7 months post-TBI
- LFPI mice had increased susceptibility to PTZ seizures

Grade 1–3 events:
- Almost all rats with rpFPI develop spontaneous chronic rhythmic (theta-alpha) patterns, focal perilesional or bilateral, 0.4–40.5 sec long, associated with behavioral arrests
- 80% of rats develop such patterns ≥5 sec long
- 100% of rats develop such patterns ≥0.8 sec long
- Their frequency increases with time | 61, 145 |

Table 1.1 (cont.)

Model	Sex, species, age	Induction method (anesthesia, method)	Gross pathology	Acute post-TBI seizure-like events and mortality	PTE rate and characteristics	References
					'Idiopathic seizures', - 3.6% of rpFPI rats (vs. 33% of 7-month-old controls) developed high amplitude sharp wave parieto-occipital discharges, 27–28 weeks post-TBI	
Controlled cortical impact model						
CCI	Male – SDR, adult	Isoflurane, CCI right parietal, 4 m/sec, 100 msec, 2.5 mm depth	- Ipsilateral necrotic cavities - Cell loss at cortex and hippocampus - Astrogliosis - Abnormal Timm staining in CCI rats	- 12.3% acute post-CCI seizures	*Monitoring done for 356–404 hr* **Video monitoring:** - 19% of CCI rats had class 3–5 seizures **Video-EEG monitoring:** - 17.5% nonconvulsive seizures with behavioral arrest - 5% had class 5 seizures - Generalized SWDs present, 8–11 Hz	71

CCI	Male – C57BL/6 mice, adult	Pentobarbital, left lateral parietotemporal craniotomy 5 mm. CCI done 45 min later (3 mm tip, 0.5 mm depth, 5 m/sec, dwell time 100 msec)	- Cortical and hippocampal injury - Hippocampal injury in 60% of CCI mice - Abnormal Timm staining in hippocampus (83%) - Increased mossy fiber sprouting in mice with spikes	- 10% acute mortality	**At 6 months post-TBI** - 9% had SRS at 6 months post-CCI - Mean SRS frequency 0.23±0.11 per day Mean SRS duration 50 ±14 sec - Mean SRS scale 3.3 ± 0.9, modified Racine scale - ~80% had epileptic spikes - None had epileptiform discharges (rhythmic transients 1–5 sec with spikes and sharps).
CCI	Male – CD-1 mice, adult	Isoflurane, left lateral craniotomy 5 mm, CCI 3 mm impact tip, 2 mm depth, 5 m/sec, 100 msec	- Cortical and hippocampal injury - Mossy fiber sprouting	- 31% acute seizures	**PTZ test, 7 months post-TBI** - CCI mice had increased susceptibility to PTZ seizures - 50% PTE - 0.27±0.11 SRS/day - 35.5±2.8 sec duration - Latency to first seizure 82.3±10.2 days

Table 1.1 (cont.)

Model	Sex, species, age	Induction method (anesthesia, method)	Gross pathology	Acute post-TBI seizure-like events and mortality	PTE rate and characteristics	References
CCI	*Male – Harlan CD-1 mice, adult*	Isoflurane, lateral craniotomy 4 mm, CCI 3 mm tip, 0.5–1 mm depth, 3.5 m/sec, 400 msec duration	- Ipsilateral cortical injury, somatosensory cortex		**Video monitoring only, starting 42 days after CCI** - Freezing, head nodding: 20% in mild CCI, 36% in severe CCI - Single forelimb myoclonus: 18% of severe CCI	[70]
CCI	*Male – C57BL/6 J mice, P21*	2,2,2-tribromoethanol ip or isoflurane, CCI **Severe**: 4.5 m/sec, 1.73 mm depth, 150 msec **Moderate**: 4 m/sec, 1.2 mm depth, 150 msec	- Astrogliosis hippocampal		- PTE rate 87% at 4–5 months (at least 1 generalized motor seizure) vs. >10% in shams - daily seizures more frequent in CCI vs. sham	[80]
Other models
Blast TBI	*Male – C57BL/6 mice, adult*	Ketamine, dexmedetomidine, blast injury, 14.6 psi, Repeated TBI 3×	Increased Iba1, tau and tau phosphonylation in the brain	- 50% acute or early seizures	**Intermittent EEG monitoring for months post-TBI** - 46% SRS, nonconvulsive	[90]

| Penetrating TBI | Male – Charles River SDR, adult | Isoflurane, Steel burr 1.5 mm diameter 1000 revolutions/min, pushed in brain 8 mm below surface; copper or stainless steel wire or nothing placed in lesion | Lesion across tract (2 mm). Rats with seizures had more extensive lesion to ventral areas, amygdala and piriform Copper wire resulted in larger lesions and discoloration with copper precipitation | **Early seizures, days 3–5 post-TBI (nonconvulsive):**
- Copper group: 70%
- Stainless steel group: 83% | - Copper group: 96% PTE, 3.6 ±0.34 seizures/day
- Steel group: 0% PTE
- Lesion only: 23% PTE
- Control: 15% PTE | 94 |

CCI: controlled cortical impact; cFPI: central fluid percussion injury; FPI: fluid percussion injury; LE: Long Evans; LFPI: lateral FPI; PTE: posttraumatic epilepsy; PTZ: pentylenetetrazol; rpFPI: rostral parasagittal FPI; SDR: Sprague Dawley rat; TBI: traumatic brain injury.

Table 1.2 Models of TBI with comorbidities

Model	Sex, species, age at TBI	Cognitive, behavioral comorbidities	References
LFPI	Rats, adult	- Visuo-spatial learning (MWM), sensorimotor deficits (beam task), anxiety (elevated plus maze) present - Cognitive deficits did not predict PTE	21, 51
LFPI	Rats, P17–19	Cognitive deficits Depression-like behavior Anxiety-like behavior Sleep abnormalities Locomotor impairment	43, 48, 146–148
cFPI	Male – SDR, adult	Locomotor deficits 4–8 days post-TBI	144
CCI	Male – SDR rats / adult	Spatial learning and memory deficits (MWM) Motor deficits	149
CCI	Female – C57BL/6 mice, adult	Persisting impairment in spatial learning (MWM) Transient motor deficits (elevated narrow beam)	150
CCI	Male – SDR rats, P28	Spatial memory deficits (MWM) Short term memory (novel object recognition) Increased impulsive-like and anti-anxiety behavior (elevated plus maze)	151
CCI	Male – SDR rats, P7 vs. P17	P7: MWM deficits on day 11 post-TBI with more severe lesions P17: MWM deficits on day 11 post-TBI with all injury severities	109
CCI	Male – C57BL/6 J Mice / P21	Hyperactivity. Spatial memory deficits Social dysfunction	80, 152

Model	Animal, age	Findings	Ref.
CCI	Male C57BL/6 mice, P21–25 vs. adult	Spatial learning deficits seen only in adult but not P21–25 injured mice (Barnes maze). No deficits in open field, light/dark test, tail suspension test found	[153]
Closed head, weight drop, impact acceleration model	SDR rats, P17	Visuospatial learning impairment (MWM). Locomotor deficits (beam balance, incline plane)	[105]
Weight drop model, closed skull	Both sexes, SDR rats, P30	Motor / balance impairment (beam walking, open field activity) – 1–2 days post-TBI. Executive functioning deficits (novel context mismatch) – 5–8 days post-TBI. Depression-like deficits (forced swim test) – 15 days post-TBI. Decreased anxiety in males (elevated plus maze) – 1 day post-TBI. Spatial learning (MWM) – 10–13 days post-TBI	[116]

CCI: controlled cortical impact; cFPI: central fluid percussion injury; LE: Long Evans; LFPI: lateral FPI; MWM: Morris water maze; PTE: posttraumatic epilepsy; P: postnatal day; PTZ: pentylenetetrazol; rpFPI: rostral parasagittal FPI; SDR: Sprague Dawley rat; TBI: traumatic brain injury.

interferon gamma (IFN-γ),[54] microglial activation and reactive astrocytosis,[52] axonal injury at white matter tracts such as the corpus callosum,[52] and decrease in protein phosphatase 2A (PP2A) activity[21] associated with overexpression of phosphorylated tau protein.[21, 57, 58]

The FPI model has been widely used as a model for PTE. The incidence of epilepsy after FPI depends on the severity, location of the injury, duration and time points used for monitoring for seizures, type of seizure-like patterns detected and the age of the animals. In studies from adult rodents that looked at EEG seizure rhythmic patterns with evolution in patterns, frequency, location, amplitude, the rate of PTE was more modest and increased with time from injury. In a longitudinal study utilizing video-EEG intermittent recordings in lateral FPI (LFPI) rats, the PTE rate was ~11% at 15–17 weeks post-injury, 30% at 7 months and ~50% at 12 months post-TBI,[59] and these seizures also included more classical motor correlates. For example, in adult male LFPI rats,[60] 50% of the animals presented focal seizures, 17% had generalized seizures and 87.5% developed late focal seizures. Similar rates ranging between 30% and 50% at 6–12 months post-TBI were also described by other groups modelling severe LFPI injury.[21, 51, 58, 60] In mice, the rate of PTE may vary according to strain. In C57BL/6S mice, 3% developed PTE till 9 months post-injury, whereas the majority (71%) developed interictal epileptic activity.[41, 44, 53] In D'Ambrosio's studies, using the rostral parasagittal FPI model in postnatal day 33–35 (P33–35, peripubertal) old rats, the reported seizure patterns consisted of focal or bilateral rhythmic activity occasionally with rhythmic spikes were described as grade 1 (focal, ipsilateral to lesion, brief), grade 2 (focal to bilateral) or grade 3 (bilateral) in up to 100% of the FPI animals by 9 weeks post-FPI.[61] Behaviorally, these patterns were associated with no or mild manifestations (freezing, facial automatisms, head nodding or myoclonus). EEG patterns described as 'idiopathic' with rhythmic spikes at the parieto-occipital regions bilaterally were also seen in older animals, 27–28 weeks post-TBI and also in 33% of controls. Table 1.1 presents a summary of studies on PTE models.

A point of caution in such studies is the detection of bursts of spike-wave discharges in the various rodent cohorts associated with freezing, immobility and often terminated with sudden movement. These may resemble the absence-type seizure patterns seen in absence epilepsy models, can be focal or bilateral and can be seen also in cohorts of experimental controls, increasing with age.[62] In an injured brain, such patterns may be altered in morphology or rate of appearance and it is highly recommended to have similarly monitored controls to establish the effect of injury on these naturally occurring patterns. Furthermore, rare occurrences of seizures in experimental controls undergoing video-EEG have been reported due to complications or predisposing conditions,[62] emphasizing the need for similar video-EEG monitoring protocols in the study controls.

Although the FPI model is an important tool for the study of PTE development and screening of pharmacological interventions with potential to act in disease-modification and prevent the development of PTE, as all models, it has some limitations. To simulate the brain injury, a craniotomy is necessary to expose the brain. This procedure itself can be potentially the cause or part of the brain injury.[54] Studies have shown that sham animals, exposed only to the craniotomy surgery, without the injury, had focal seizure after the procedure.[60] In the same way, increase in cytokines, KC-GRO (growth-regulated oncogenes (GRO) / keratinocyte chemoattractant (KC)) and IFN-γ have been reported in sham animals compared to naïve.[54, 59, 63] Optimization of the conditions for the induction of FPI injury is needed in each laboratory to ensure that the acute outcomes are equivalent to parameters used for the desired injury severity. This model has a high incidence of acute mortality post-injury, about 30% when severe, requiring a high number of animals to achieve power for statistical analyses.[54, 59, 63]

Controlled Cortical Impact (CCI) Model

The controlled cortical impact (CCI)[64] model was developed in the 1980s to simulate human closed-head TBI in the ferret and create a test to determine changes in brain tissue after a direct mechanical deformation,[65, 66] and it is widely used especially in rodents, generating cortical and hippocampal focal lesions.[53, 54, 67-73] The CCI consists in impacting the cortical area through a stroke-constrained pneumatic impactor. This can be done either through a pre-existing craniotomy on an intact dura,[65] or by impacting the intact skull.[66] The tip of the impactor can vary in size and geometry, and CCI devices allow control of the speed, depth and duration of impact.[66] All those parameters can determine the severity of the trauma, underlying pathology and the subsequent rate of PTE; it is therefore important to standardize these conditions in each laboratory when establishing the model.

Similar to the FPI, the CCI model leads to memory and learning deficits,[67-69, 72] dysfunction in the motor and sensory systems,[54, 69] and also affects psychosocial-related behaviors[69] (Table 1.2). In pediatric CCI studies, cognitive impairment and sensori-motor deficits along with anxiety-like behaviors even 2 months after injury are typical in P17 rats that have been subjected to CCI. Neuronal reorganization and alterations in white matter may also ensue.[74, 75] Recently, P21 mice were exposed to CCI, which led to neuropathological characteristics consistent with PTE, like mossy fiber sprouting and neuroinflammation resulting in cortical atrophy and hippocampal sclerosis. These mice also exhibited behavioral abnormalities such as hyperactivity, social impairment and memory deficits.[76-79] In addition to that there was a strong increase in vulnerability to provoked seizures in response to intraperitoneal (i.p.) pentylenetetrazole (PTZ, $GABA_A$ receptor antagonist) administration, as early as 2 weeks post-TBI and persisting until at least 6 months later. Furthermore, more than 87% of the CCI mice had at least one generalized motor seizure during a 7-day video EEG recording at 4–5 months post-injury.[6, 80]

The rate of PTE post-CCI varies across studies, ranging between 9% and 50% depending on the injury severity, location, strain and criteria for seizure detection[53, 69, 71] (Table 1.1). As in the FPI model, the rate of interictal epileptic discharges is significantly higher, up to 82%.[53, 69] The CCI model is widely used, has similarly high mortality as the LFPI model of severe TBI (around 30% in severe TBI),[54] and there is no injury parameter standardization.[66]

Blast-induced Traumatic Brain Injury (bTBI) Model

An explosion causes a high speed blast wave. When this blast wave hits one's body it is absorbed and propagated causing widespread damage, including to the brain.[81] TBI caused by blast can be correlated to three different events: primary blast injury – result of the wave air dislocation; secondary blast injury – impact of fragments due to the explosion; tertiary blast injury – when one is thrown away by the blast.[82] Some experiments with animal models are done in free-field blast, where real explosives can be used in large animals as pigs and sheep.[17] For rodents, usually a long metal blast tube with explosives is used to generate the blast wave and the animal is positioned in a specific distance of the explosion.[82] The closer the explosion focus is, the higher is the severity and mortality of the model.[83]

The bTBI is not as widely studied as the FPI or CCI and may carry more inherent variability in the injury, both within and outside the brain, which may complicate the study design. However, it is a more realistic model for military field-based TBI caused by explosions. Similar to the other TBI models, it may result in inflammatory responses in the brain, elevation in glial fibrillary acidic protein (GFAP) in the ventral hippocampus, prefrontal cortex and amygdala.[84] Levels of IFN-γ and interleukin-6 (IL-6) were increased in amygdala and ventral hippocampus.[84, 85] After bTBI, rats had increase in anxiety-like behaviour,[84, 86–88] and elevated levels of serum corticosterone[84] as well as depression-like behaviors and cognitive impairments.[84, 86–89] Spontaneous seizures have been described as more frequent in models of repeated (3×) bTBI than in single bTBI[90] (Table 1.1).

Penetrating Brain Injury Model

Penetrating brain injury is caused by an object that penetrates the brain, for example, a gun bullet. This is the injury type with the higher risk of PTE development, especially if pieces of bone or foreign fragments are retained inside the brain.[17] Besides the fragments in the brain, the bullet also makes a cavity larger than its own size. In order to simulate the penetrating ballistic-like brain injury, some studies were done using a custom probe inserted in the animal's brain. The probe is connected to an elastic balloon on the tip that is quickly inflated inside the brain making thus the cavity similar to a bullet's penetration.[91–93]

Anatomical and physiological changes due to the probe penetration and inflammation in the rat's brain are seen. Intracranial hemorrhage and lesion size have been correlated to the injury severity as shown by increase in hemispheric swelling due to rise in intracranial pressure.[93] Penetrating brain injury also leads to impairment in sensorimotor skills and spatial learning deficits in rats.[92, 93] Likewise, this model caused incidence of nonconvulsive seizures and periodic epileptiform discharges, and both were positively correlated with the severity of the injury.[91]

The limitation of using the probe is that it does not mimic the penetration of fragments of bone or pieces of the penetrating object. To overcome this, a new model was developed using a high speed drill, whereby a 1-mm diameter steel burr was pushed through the exposed skull into the brain, from the dorsal cortex to the ventral hippocampus, and the fragments were not removed.[94] Interestingly, the injured animals that received copper wire in the lesion were more likely to develop epilepsy (96% vs. 15% of the steel injured rats).[94] Copper is present in bullets, suggesting that it may be an important inducer of PTE development after gunshot wounds.[94]

Weight-drop Models

Different weight-drop models have been developed over the years in rats and mice and are induced by a guided weight that is released to impact the animal's head. Feeney's model was the first to be developed and requires a craniotomy to expose the dura mater and mainly provokes a focal injury.[4] The animal is positioned under a cylinder that contains a weight and a footplate. The weight is released and strikes the footplate that goes over the exposed intact dura, generating the brain injury.[95] This trauma caused cortical contusion and white matter hemorrhage which progresses to a necrotic cavity that can expand over the time.[95–97]

The Marmarou's impact acceleration model does not require a craniotomy but only a surgical procedure to expose the skull. A metal disk is glued on the exposed skull midline, between bregma and lambda, and acts as a helmet avoiding bone fracture. The animal is placed with the disc attached on a foam platform and a brass weight is released inside a Plexiglas tube on the disk causing a diffuse axonal injury.[98] This type of injury is usually seen after falls or car accidents.[4] Motor and cognitive impairments are observed after trauma.[99, 100] Anatomical diffuse damage can be seen in axonal and dendritic structures, as well as injury in microvasculature.[101] The limitations of these models are that there is a high variability of severity and the mortality is relatively high in severe injury, and it is caused basically by respiratory depression.[4]

Shohami's model also consists of a focal closed-head injury and does not require a craniotomy. In this model, an incision is made to expose the skull and then a weight is released to fall upon one side of the unprotected rodent's skull.[102] The trauma caused by the weight drop leads to motor function, memory deficits, cerebral edema, hippocampal neuronal death and breakdown of the blood–brain barrier (BBB) in the mouse brain.[103, 104] In this model, the device is easy to operate, however, it is not highly reproducible.[4]

In the pediatric version of the weight drop model, a helmet is often utilized so as to prevent penetration and later skull fractures, which are very common in small and young animals after injury.[95, 98] Severe injury in this model can also mimic the extended swelling and neurocognitive impairment that is quite often seen in brain-injured children.[105–107] Specifically, injury of P17 animals can lead to vestibulomotor deficit up to 10 days post-TBI, as well as remarkable axonal injury and astrogliosis and deficits in the Morris Water Maze test of visuospatial learning and memory, 3 months after the trauma[108, 109] (Table 1.2).

TBI-related Brain Pathologies, Age Dependence and Relevance to PTE

TBI causes multifaceted and multifocal pathologies in the brain that may progress or evolve with time, setting the stage for the development of resultant neurological, functional deficits or epileptogenesis. Immediate changes include the structural lesions caused by TBI: skull fracture, dura deficits, axonal injuries and cell loss, disruption of the integrity of extracellular matrix and neurovascular units resulting in BBB disruption, hemorrhages and edema. The acute post-traumatic seizures, when present, or systemic disorders, such as hypoxia or metabolic changes during the acute and subacute critical post-TBI periods, may further exacerbate these pathologies. The subsequent cellular or molecular changes include cell proliferation (including neurogenesis), gliosis, synaptic remodeling and inflammation that further modify the structural and functional disturbances that define the long-term TBI outcomes. Both clinical and preclinical studies have suggested that these effects may depend upon the severity and nature of the TBI but also may be further modified by biological factors, such as age or sex. A limitation for across age comparisons stems from the striking anatomical differences (skull and brain size, skull thickness and integrity) that challenge the comparisons of the strength and propagation routes of the applied pressure pulses or the equivalency of other TBI induction methods. Regardless, we will discuss here selected examples of TBI-related pathologies and their potential relevance to long-term TBI outcomes, including PTE. In addition, in Table 1.3 we summarize the preclinical trials testing new treatments to modify PTE rate and severity.

Table 1.3 Preclinical trials for effects on spontaneous seizures in PTE models

Treatment	Mechanism	Model	Effects on seizures	References
Atipemazole	α2 adrenergic antagonist	LFPI, adult rats	No effect on spontaneous seizures Reduces PTZ seizure susceptibility	154
Ceftriaxone	Antibiotic, increases expression of glutamate transporter GLT-1	LFPI, adult rats	Reduced cumulative seizure duration 12 weeks post-TBI	155
Focal cooling	Focal cooling 0.5–2°C	rpFPI, P32–36 rats	Abolished ictal activity up to 10 weeks post-TBI Ictal events: rhythmic spike waves with freeze-like arrest	156
Rapamycin	mTOR inhibition	CCI, adult CD1 mice	Reduced PTE rate at 4 months post-CCI (by video-EEG monitoring)	69
Rapamycin	mTOR inhibition	CCI, adult CD1 mice	No effect on behavioral seizures (visual monitoring only)	136
Sodium selenate	Protein phosphatase 2A activator	LFPI, adult rats	Reduced seizure frequency during and after treatment	58
Kineret	Interleukin 1 receptor antagonist	CCI, P21 C57BL/6 J mice	No effects on spontaneous seizures, reduced PTZ seizure susceptibility	80

The table is modified version of Table 1 in Saletti et al. (2019)[6] and reproduced with permission from Elsevier.
CCI: controlled cortical impact; LFPI: lateral FPI; P: postnatal day; PTE: posttraumatic epilepsy; PTZ: pentylenetetrazol; rpFPI: rostral parasagittal FPI; TBI: traumatic brain injury.

TBI can increase neurogenesis in specific brain regions, such as the subventricular zone of the lateral ventricles and the dentate gyrus.[110] Using the LFPI model, both the number of newborn cells at the subgranular zone of dentate gyrus as well as their differentiation to neurons was greater in rats injured at P18 (juvenile) than in adulthood.[111] Similarly, CCI induced a stronger proliferative response ipsilateral to the lesion, when injury was induced at P6, P11 or P17 compared to adulthood.[112] Whether early increase in post-TBI neurogenesis favors recovery or promotes epileptogenesis has been debated. A recent study suggested that early neurogenesis in the LFPI model in P23–25 Wistar rats promotes excitability and increases seizure susceptibility to induced seizures post-TBI.[113]

The formation of new dendritic arbors, synapses and synaptic pruning, that is the selective retention of synapses that are functionally important and useful, are critical steps for the normal brain development. Injuries may damage axonal and synaptic connections or may create aberrant connections that may contribute to epileptogenesis or comorbidogenesis. In CCI-injured adult rats, a 60% loss of synapses in the CA1 sector of the hippocampus was observed at 2 days post-CCI and a gradual, but partial recovery was noted till 60 days post-CCI.[114] However, this post-TBI partial recovery in synaptogenesis did not translate in to improved spatial learning. Further, a characteristic pathology of hippocampal epileptogenesis (aberrant mossy fiber sprouting at the inner molecular layer) was reported in all CCI-injured adult rats.[71] Age-dependent vulnerability to injury has been reported in the CCI model, whereby the morphology and complexity of dendrites was not affected after CCI in P7 rats as opposed to P17 and P30 rats, in which region-specific changes were observed.[115–117] Other studies recorded a higher rate of synaptic sprouting in P35 rats compared to adult rats[118] as well as plastic reorganization of circuitry in the injured brain cortex and hippocampus.[75] This circuitry reorganization has been correlated with gradual lesion extension and transient behavioral phenotypes, suggesting the implication of post-traumatic plasticity to dysfunctional neuronal networks leading to proneness to seizures.[119]

Inflammatory signaling pathways have attracted attention for their potential role for epileptogenesis under different settings, including TBI [6, 120, 121] (Table 1.1, Table 1.3). It has been proposed that the developing brain elicits more robust inflammatory response in response to TBI, greater disruption of BBB and is less capable in counterbalancing oxidative stress or detoxifying free iron after TBI induced bleeding.[120] In the CCI model, P21 C57BL/6 mice showed more pronounced acute and more prolonged cortical infiltration by CD45+ leukocytes or GR−1+ granulocytes in the developing brain than in the adult brain. Cortical volume loss was more pronounced acutely in adults but showed progressive deterioration in the injured P21 mice.[122] Increased levels of Interleukin 1β (IL-1β) levels were observed in P21 mice in the cortex, hippocampus and serum during the first days after TBI; treatment with IL-1 receptor antagonist (IL-1Ra) improved spatial memory and susceptibility to evoked seizures, although no significant effect was seen over spontaneous seizures[80] (Table 1.3).

The brain is highly susceptible to oxidative damage because of its high rate of oxidative activity and the relatively low antioxidant capacity. Enzymes such as superoxide dismutase (SOD), catalase and glutathione peroxidase act against the production of reactive oxygen species (ROS). In mice, catalase, total SOD and total glutathione peroxidase enzyme activities increase from the embryonic to the early postnatal (P1) period and either decline (total SOD, total glutathione peroxidase activity) or gradually increase till P21.[123] In rats, the activity of these enzymes also increases between the embryonic to early postnatal days, but the trajectory of these changes differs thereafter, with SOD and glutathione peroxidase activities increasing through adulthood and catalase activity decreasing between P10 and adulthood.[124–126] These suggest age- and possibly species-specific responses to insults that produce oxidative stress, such as TBI.

Recently, research has been focused on the effect TBI can have on cerebral metabolism mainly in the developing brain. Cerebral metabolic abnormalities in infants and children after closed head injury have been linked to poor neurodevelopmental outcomes.[127, 128] A decrease in cerebral glucose metabolism has been described in P17–21 rats after CCI.[129–131] An age-dependent switch from ketones to glucose as the main fuel source of brain probably contributes to the flexibility of the developing brain to metabolic disruption. Pre-weanling and even peripubertal rodents (~P35) have a better capacity for ketone uptake and metabolism than the adult animals, which possibly adds to the better metabolic response and neurochemical balance in the immature brain after injury.[132, 133] A ketogenic diet has been tried in adult LFPI-injured rats and increased the threshold for flurothyl induced seizures but has not been tested on spontaneous seizures.[134]

There are several pathologies and pathways that have been investigated for their role in PTE epileptogenesis and post-TBI sequelae. The mechanistic target of rapamycin (mTOR) pathway is a critical hub in many epileptogenic pathways and has shown disease modifying effects in several models of epilepsy.[135] In the CCI model, rapamycin has reduced the rate of PTE in adult mice in a study using video-EEG recordings but did not show efficacy in a trial using only visual monitoring for seizures.[69, 136] Earlier studies, in the closed head weight drop model, showed functional and behavioral improvement with rapamycin.[137]

Traumatic brain hemorrhage is a well-known risk factor for the development of PTE, both due to direct structural lesions but also due to iron toxicity and/or accumulation and production of free radicals.[6] Ferric chloride is a known precipitant of focal epileptogenesis when injected in the sensorimotor cortex.[138] An intracortical iron injection TBI model has been developed and more excitatory neurotransmitters were reported in the brain of rats with seizures compared to those that did not manifest seizures.[139] Since TBI can also result from trauma that includes introduction of metals in the brain, the role of metals has been investigated. Copper, for example, has been proposed as more epileptogenic than stainless steel in a penetrating injury TBI model[94] (Table 1.1).

The hyperphosphorylation of tau protein, an integral pathology in many neurodegenerative disorders, post-traumatic encephalopathy and some epilepsies, has attracted a lot of interest for its potential contribution to both post-TBI comorbidities and PTE.[2] The first preclinical studies demonstrated promising effects of drugs that reduce hyperphosphorylated tau in the LFPI model, in regards to ameliorating spontaneous seizures and post-TBI pathologies.[21, 58] Pathological hyperphosphorylation of tau has been demonstrated in several models of TBI and remains an interesting pathology for future studies.[140]

The Operation Brain Trauma Therapy (OBTT), a multicenter preclinical consortium for the screening for treatments and biomarkers has investigated several candidate treatments for their effect in various TBI models, on neurological, cognitive and histology outcomes, as well as on serum biomarkers, like GFAP (glial fibrillary astrocytic protein) and UCH-L1 (ubiquitin carboxy-terminal hydrolase-L1).[141] Among the drugs with the best profile included levetiracetam, which improved cognitive function in the LFPI and CCI models with excellent tolerability.[141] Levetiracetam is commonly given during the acute phase of severe TBI patients to prevent early seizures and consequent harmful complications, although there is no evidence of antiepileptogenic effect for these drugs, preclinical studies indicated some benefit, possibly attributed to the antiseizure effect and reduction of inflammation.

There is currently no evidence for validated antiepileptogenic treatment in TBI. Several treatments have been tested preclinically (Table 1.3) though validation through additional studies needs to be done. The Epilepsy Bioinformatics Study for Antiepileptogenic Therapy, EpiBioS4Rx, is an National Institute of Neurological Disorders and Stroke (NINDS) funded international preclinical and clinical multicenter without walls that aims to create a platform for the identification, validation and translation of new treatments to prevent PTE through the use of biomarkers and rigorous multicenter studies in the LFPI model.[142, 143]

Conclusions

Significant progress has been achieved through the development and use of animal models in elucidating mechanisms for post-TBI pathologies, epilepsy and comorbidities, and testing new treatments. A great challenge in this endeavor is the inherent variability of pathology (cause, type, location, multifocality, nature of pathological changes) seen in TBI, in humans that make it challenging to extrapolate and generalize the findings and prognosis. Animal models have tried to standardize, to some extent, this variability, although all models exhibit significant challenges in standardizing the induced injury. Models have been useful in proposing targets, biomarkers and candidate treatments for TBI and PTE. There is a significant need for agreement in the community on best measurements and standardization methods as well as approaches that would help translate findings from animals and humans. Efforts to promote these discussions and accelerate progress are ongoing through collaborations of funders, investigators and professional organizations, and through the development of common data elements to improve reporting and comparison of data. A transformation in the way preclinical research is done has been the creation of multicenter consortia, preclinical and clinical, for example, EpiBioS4Rx, OBTT or the TBI initiative of CURE (Citizens United for Research in Epilepsy), funded by the US Department of Defense, that promises to change management of individuals with TBI and PTE by improving our ability to prognosticate, select candidates for best treatments and offer better therapies.

Acknowledgements

PGS, AMK, MM have no conflicts of interest.

ASG acknowledges grant support by NINDS RO1 NS091170, the NINDS Center without WallsU54 NS100064 (EpiBioS4Rx), the United States Department of Defense (W81XWH-18-1-0612 W81XWH-13–1-0180), and American Epilepsy Society (seed grant) research funding from the Heffer Family, the Segal Family Foundations and the Abbe Goldstein/Joshua Lurie, and Laurie Marsh/Dan Levitz families. ASG has received royalties for publications from Elsevier Medlink and Morgan & Claypool, and a one-time honorarium for participation at a scientific advisory board for Eisai and is a Editor-in-Chief at *Epilepsia Open* but has no conflicts in regards to this chapter.

References

1. Centers for Disease Control and Prevention. Traumatic Brain Injury & Concussion 2019. Available from: www.cdc.gov/traumaticbraininjury/index.html.

2. I. Ali, J.C. Silva, S. Liu, et al. Targeting neurodegeneration to prevent post-traumatic epilepsy. *Neurobiol Dis* 2019;123:100–9.

3. R.F. Hunt, J.A. Boychuk, B.N. Smith. Neural circuit mechanisms of post-traumatic epilepsy. *Front Cell Neurosci* 2013;7:89.

4. Y. Xiong, A. Mahmood, M. Chopp. Animal models of traumatic brain injury. *Nat Rev Neurosci* 2013;14(2):128–42.

5. C.C. Giza, R.B. Mink, A. Madikians. Pediatric traumatic brain injury: not just little adults. *Curr Op Crit Care* 2007;13(2):143–52.

6. P.G. Saletti, I. Ali, P.M. Casillas-Espinosa, et al. In search of antiepileptogenic treatments for post-traumatic epilepsy. *Neurobiol Dis* 2019;123:86–99.

7. J. Christensen. Traumatic brain injury: risks of epilepsy and implications for medicolegal assessment. *Epilepsia* 2012;53 Suppl 4:43–7.

8. J. Christensen, M.G. Pedersen, C.B. Pedersen, P. Sidenius, J. Olsen, M. Vestergaard. Long-term risk of epilepsy after traumatic brain injury in children and young adults: a population-based cohort study. *Lancet* 2009;373(9669):1105–10.

9. R.S. Fisher, C. Acevedo, A. Arzimanoglou, et al. ILAE official report: a practical clinical definition of epilepsy. *Epilepsia* 2014;55(4):475–82.

10. I.E. Scheffer, J. French, E. Hirsch, et al. Classification of the epilepsies: New concepts for discussion and debate-Special report of the ILAE Classification Task Force of the Commission for Classification and Terminology. *Epilepsia Open* 2016;1(1–2):37–44.

11. K. Ding, P.K. Gupta, R. Diaz-Arrastia. Epilepsy after traumatic brain injury. In: Laskowitz D, Grant G, eds. *Translational Research in Traumatic Brain Injury. Frontiers in Neuroscience.* Boca Raton (FL): CRC Press/Taylor and Francis Group;2016.

12. J. Englander, T. Bushnik, J.M. Wright, L. Jamison, T.T. Duong. Mortality in late post-traumatic seizures. *J Neurotrauma* 2009;26(9):1471–7.

13. A. Agrawal, J. Timothy, L. Pandit, M. Manju. Post-traumatic epilepsy: an overview. *Clin Neurol Neurosurg* 2006;108(5):433–9.

14. R. D'Ambrosio, E. Perucca. Epilepsy after head injury. *Curr Opin Neurol* 2004;17(6):731–5.

15. T. Xu, X. Yu, S. Ou, et al. Risk factors for posttraumatic epilepsy: A systematic review and meta-analysis. *Epilepsy Behav* 2017;67:1–6.

16. M.A. Tubi, E. Lutkenhoff, M.B. Blanco, et al. Early seizures and temporal lobe trauma predict post-traumatic epilepsy: A longitudinal study. *Neurobiol Dis* 2019;123:115–21.

17. R.D. Brady, P.M. Casillas-Espinosa, D.V. Agoston, et al. Modelling traumatic brain injury and posttraumatic epilepsy in rodents. *Neurobiol Dis* 2019;123:8–19.

18. V.P. Johnstone, D.K. Wright, K. Wong, T.J. O'Brien, R. Rajan, S.R. Shultz. Experimental traumatic brain injury results in long-term recovery of functional responsiveness in sensory cortex but persisting structural changes and sensorimotor, cognitive, and emotional deficits. *J Neurotrauma* 2015;32(17):1333–46.

19. N.C. Jones, L. Cardamone, J.P. Williams, M.R. Salzberg, D. Myers, T.J. O'Brien. Experimental traumatic brain injury induces a pervasive hyperanxious phenotype in rats. *J Neurotrauma* 2008;25(11):1367–74.

20. K.M. Rodgers, Y.K. Deming, F.M. Bercum, et al. Reversal of established traumatic brain injury-induced, anxiety-like behavior in rats after delayed, post-injury neuroimmune suppression. *J Neurotrauma* 2014;31(5):487–97.

21. S.R. Shultz, D.K. Wright, P. Zheng, et al. Sodium selenate reduces hyperphosphorylated tau and improves outcomes after traumatic brain injury. *Brain* 2015;138(5):1297–313.

22. M.H. Beauchamp, V. Anderson. Cognitive and psychopathological sequelae of pediatric traumatic brain injury. In: Dulac O., Lassonde M., Sarnat H.B., eds. *Handbook of Clinical Neurology.* Philadelphia, PA: Elsevier, 2013; 112:913–20.

23. V.A. Anderson, M.M. Spencer-Smith, L. Coleman, et al. Predicting neurocognitive and behavioural outcome after early brain insult. *Developmental Medicine and Child Neurology* 2014;56 (4):329–36.

24. J. Luo, A. Nguyen, S. Villeda, et al. Long-term cognitive impairments and pathological alterations in a mouse model of repetitive mild traumatic brain injury. *Front Neurol* 2014;5:12.

25. M.M. Muccigrosso, J. Ford, B. Benner, et al. Cognitive deficits develop 1 month after diffuse brain injury and are exaggerated by microglia-associated reactivity to peripheral immune challenge. *Brain Behav Immun* 2016;54:95–109.

26. M. Ogier, A. Belmeguenai, T. Lieutaud, et al. Cognitive deficits and inflammatory response resulting from mild-to-moderate traumatic brain injury in rats are exacerbated by repeated pre-exposure to an innate stress stimulus. *J Neurotrauma* 2017;34(8):1645–57.

27. R.J. Castriotta, M.C. Wilde, J.M. Lai, S. Atanasov, B.E. Masel, S.T. Kuna. Prevalence and consequences of sleep disorders in traumatic brain injury. *J Clin Sleep Med* 2007;3(4):349–56.

28. B.C. Vos, K. Nieuwenhuijsen, J.K. Sluiter. Consequences of traumatic brain injury in professional american football players: A systematic review of the literature. *Clin J Sport Med* 2018;28(2):91–9.

29. B.D. Semple, A. Zamani, G. Rayner, S. R. Shultz, N.C. Jones. Affective, neurocognitive and psychosocial disorders associated with traumatic brain injury and post-traumatic epilepsy. *Neurobiol Dis* 2019;123:27–41.

30. F.E. Dudek, K.J. Staley. The time course of acquired epilepsy: implications for therapeutic intervention to suppress epileptogenesis. *Neurosci Lett* 2011;497 (3):240–6.

31. P. Klein, R. Dingledine, E. Aronica, et al. Commonalities in epileptogenic processes from different acute brain insults: Do they translate? *Epilepsia* 2018;59(1):37–66.

32. O. Akman, S.L. Moshe, A.S. Galanopoulou. Sex-specific consequences of early life seizures. *Neurobiol Dis* 2014;72 Pt B:153–66.

33. A.S. Galanopoulou, S.L. Moshe. In search of epilepsy biomarkers in the immature brain: goals, challenges and strategies. *Biomark Med* 2011;5(5):615–28.

34. A.M. Katsarou, S.L. Moshe, A.S. Galanopoulou. Interneuronopathies and their role in early life epilepsies and neurodevelopmental disorders. *Epilepsia Open* 2017;2(3):284–306.

35. A.M. Katsarou, A.S. Galanopoulou, S.L. Moshe. Epileptogenesis in neonatal brain. *Semin Fetal Neonatal Med* 2018;23 (3):159–67.

36. A. Gottlieb, I. Keydar, H.T. Epstein. Rodent brain growth stages: an analytical review. *Biol Neonate* 1977;32(3–4):166–76.

37. J. Dobbing, J. Sands. Comparative aspects of the brain growth spurt. *Early Human Development* 1979;3:79–83.

38. S. Avishai-Eliner, K.L. Brunson, C.A. Sandman, T.Z. Baram. Stressed-out, or in (utero)? *Trends in Neurosciences* 2002;25(10):518–24.

39. H.J. Romijn, M.A. Hofman, A. Gramsbergen. At what age is the developing cerebral cortex of the rat comparable to that of the full-term newborn human baby? *Early Human Development* 1991;26(1):61–7.

40. B.D. Semple, K. Blomgren, K. Gimlin, D.M. Ferriero, L.J. Noble-Haeusslein. Brain development in rodents and humans: Identifying benchmarks of maturation and

vulnerability to injury across species. *Progress in Neurobiology* 2013;106(7):1–16.

41. M.L. Prins, D.A. Hovda. Developing experimental models to address traumatic brain injury in children. *J Neurotrauma* 2003;20(2):123–37.

42. T.K. McIntosh, R. Vink, L. Noble, et al. Traumatic brain injury in the rat: characterization of a lateral fluid-percussion model. *Neuroscience* 1989;28(1):233–44.

43. M.L. Prins, S.M. Lee, C.L. Cheng, D.P. Becker, D.A. Hovda. Fluid percussion brain injury in the developing and adult rat: a comparative study of mortality, morphology, intracranial pressure and mean arterial blood pressure. *Brain Res Developmental Brain Res* 1996;95 (2):272–82.

44. W.M. Armstead, C.D. Kurth. Different cerebral hemodynamic responses following fluid percussion brain injury in the newborn and juvenile pig. *J Neurotrauma* 1994;11(5):487–97.

45. S.L. Aungst, S.V. Kabadi, S.M. Thompson, B.A. Stoica, A.I. Faden. Repeated mild traumatic brain injury causes chronic neuroinflammation, changes in hippocampal synaptic plasticity, and associated cognitive deficits. *J Cereb Blood Flow Metab* 2014;34(7):1223–32.

46. F. Bao, S.R. Shultz, J.D. Hepburn, et al. A CD11d monoclonal antibody treatment reduces tissue injury and improves neurological outcome after fluid percussion brain injury in rats. *J Neurotrauma* 2012;29(14):2375–92.

47. A.L. DeRoss, J.E. Adams, D.W. Vane, S.J. Russell, A.M. Terella, S.L. Wald. Multiple head injuries in rats: effects on behavior. *J Trauma* 2002;52(4):708–14.

48. G.G. Gurkoff, C.C. Giza, D.A. Hovda. Lateral fluid percussion injury in the developing rat causes an acute, mild behavioral dysfunction in the absence of significant cell death. *Brain Res* 2006;1077 (1):24–36.

49. N.M. Hayward, R. Immonen, P.I. Tuunanen, X.E. Ndode-Ekane, O. Grohn, A. Pitkanen. Association of chronic vascular changes with functional outcome after traumatic brain injury in rats. *J Neurotrauma* 2010;27(12):2203–19.

50. S.R. Shultz, F. Bao, V. Omana, C. Chiu, A. Brown, D.P. Cain. Repeated mild lateral fluid percussion brain injury in the rat causes cumulative long-term behavioral impairments, neuroinflammation, and cortical loss in an animal model of repeated concussion. *J Neurotrauma* 2012;29 (2):281–94.

51. S.R. Shultz, L. Cardamone, Y.R. Liu, et al. Can structural or functional changes following traumatic brain injury in the rat predict epileptic outcome? *Epilepsia* 2013;54(7):1240–50.

52. S.R. Shultz, D.F. MacFabe, K.A. Foley, R. Taylor, D.P. Cain. A single mild fluid percussion injury induces short-term behavioral and neuropathological changes in the Long-Evans rat: support for an animal model of concussion. *Behav Brain Res* 2011;224(2):326–35.

53. T. Bolkvadze, A. Pitkanen. Development of post-traumatic epilepsy after controlled cortical impact and lateral fluid-percussion-induced brain injury in the mouse. *J Neurotrauma* 2012;29 (5):789–812.

54. J.T. Cole, A. Yarnell, W.S. Kean, et al. Craniotomy: true sham for traumatic brain injury, or a sham of a sham? *J Neurotrauma* 2011;28(3):359–69.

55. V.P.A. Johnstone, S.R. Shultz, E.B. Yan, T.J. O'Brien, R. Rajan. The acute phase of mild traumatic brain injury is characterized by a distance-dependent neuronal hypoactivity. *J Neurotraum* 2014;31(22):1881–95.

56. M.D. Skopin, S.V. Kabadi, S.S. Viechweg, J.A. Mong, A.I. Faden. Chronic decrease in wakefulness and disruption of sleep-wake behavior after experimental traumatic brain injury. *J Neurotrauma* 2015;32 (5):289–96.

57. N.C. Jones, T. Nguyen, N.M. Corcoran, et al. Targeting hyperphosphorylated tau with sodium selenate suppresses seizures in rodent models. *Neurobiol Dis* 2012;45 (3):897–901.

58. S.J. Liu, P. Zheng, D.K. Wright, et al. Sodium selenate retards epileptogenesis in acquired epilepsy models reversing changes in protein phosphatase 2A and hyperphosphorylated tau. *Brain* 2016;139 (7):1919–38.

59. I. Kharatishvili, J.P. Nissinen, T.K. McIntosh, A. Pitkanen. A model of posttraumatic epilepsy induced by lateral fluid-percussion brain injury in rats. *Neuroscience* 2006;140(2):685–97.

60. A.Y. Reid, A. Bragin, C.C. Giza, R.J. Staba, J. Engel, Jr. The progression of electrophysiologic abnormalities during epileptogenesis after experimental traumatic brain injury. *Epilepsia* 2016;57 (10):1558–67.

61. R. D'Ambrosio, J.S. Fender, J.P. Fairbanks, et al. Progression from frontal-parietal to mesial-temporal epilepsy after fluid percussion injury in the rat. *Brain* 2005;128:174–88.

62. S.D. Kadam, R. D'Ambrosio, V. Duveau, et al. Methodological standards and interpretation of video-electroencephalography in adult control rodents. A TASK1-WG1 report of the AES/ILAE Translational Task Force of the ILAE. *Epilepsia* 2017;58 Suppl 4:10–27.

63. I. Kharatishvili, R. Immonen, O. Grohn, A. Pitkanen. Quantitative diffusion MRI of hippocampus as a surrogate marker for post-traumatic epileptogenesis. *Brain* 2007;130:3155–68.

64. F. Rodriguez Lucci, M. Alet, S.F. Ameriso. [Post-stroke epilepsy]. *Medicina (B Aires).* 2018;78(2):86–90.

65. J.W. Lighthall. Controlled cortical impact: a new experimental brain injury model. *J Neurotrauma* 1988;5(1):1–15.

66. N.D. Osier, C.E. Dixon. The controlled cortical impact model: applications, considerations for researchers, and future directions. *Front Neurol* 2016;7:134.

67. I. Cernak. Animal models of head trauma. *NeuroRx* 2005;2(3):410–22.

68. G.B. Fox, L. Fan, R.A. Levasseur, A. I. Faden. Sustained sensory/motor and cognitive deficits with neuronal apoptosis following controlled cortical impact brain injury in the mouse. *J Neurotrauma* 1998;15(8):599–614.

69. D. Guo, L. Zeng, D.L. Brody, M. Wong. Rapamycin attenuates the development of posttraumatic epilepsy in a mouse model of traumatic brain injury. *PLoS One* 2013;8 (5):e64078.

70. R.F. Hunt, S.W. Scheff, B.N. Smith. Posttraumatic epilepsy after controlled cortical impact injury in mice. *Exp Neurol* 2009;215(2):243–52.

71. K.M. Kelly, E.R. Miller, E. Lepsveridze, E.A. Kharlamov, Z. McHedlishvili. Posttraumatic seizures and epilepsy in adult rats after controlled cortical impact. *Epilepsy Res* 2015;117:104–16.

72. S.W. Scheff, S.A. Baldwin, R.W. Brown, P.J. Kraemer. Morris water maze deficits in rats following traumatic brain injury: lateral controlled cortical impact. *J Neurotrauma* 1997;14(9):615–27.

73. N.D. Osier, J.R. Korpon, C.E. Dixon. Frontiers in neuroengineering. controlled cortical impact model. In: Kobeissy FH, editor. *Brain Neurotrauma: Molecular, Neuropsychological, and Rehabilitation Aspects.* Boca Raton (FL): CRC Press, Taylor & Francis Group, LLC.; 2015.

74. D.O. Ajao, V. Pop, J.E. Kamper, et al. Traumatic brain injury in young rats leads to progressive behavioral deficits coincident with altered tissue properties in adulthood. *J Neurotrauma* 2012;29 (11):2060–74.

75. J.P. Card, D.J. Santone, Jr., M.Y. Gluhovsky, P.D. Adelson. Plastic reorganization of hippocampal and neocortical circuitry in experimental traumatic brain injury in the immature rat. *J Neurotrauma* 2005;22(9):989–1002.

76. B.D. Semple, S.A. Canchola, L.J. Noble-Haeusslein. Deficits in social behavior emerge during development after pediatric traumatic brain injury in mice. *J Neurotrauma* 2012;29(17):2672–83.

77. B.D. Semple, L.J. Noble-Haeusslein, Y. Jun Kwon, et al. Sociosexual and communication deficits after traumatic

injury to the developing murine brain. *PLoS One* 2014;9(8):e103386.

78. W. Tong, T. Igarashi, D.M. Ferriero, L.J. Noble. Traumatic brain injury in the immature mouse brain: characterization of regional vulnerability. *Exp Neurol* 2002;176 (1):105–16.

79. R. Pullela, J. Raber, T. Pfankuch, et al. Traumatic injury to the immature brain results in progressive neuronal loss, hyperactivity and delayed cognitive impairments. *Developmental Neurosci* 2006;28(4–5):396–409.

80. B.D. Semple, T.J. O'Brien, K. Gimlin, et al. Interleukin-1 receptor in seizure susceptibility after traumatic injury to the pediatric brain. *J Neurosci* 2017;37 (33):7864–77.

81. G.A. Elder, E.M. Mitsis, S.T. Ahlers, A. Cristian. Blast-induced mild traumatic brain injury. *Psychiatr Clin North Am.* 2010;33(4):757–81.

82. M. Risling, S. Plantman, M. Angeria, et al. Mechanisms of blast induced brain injuries, experimental studies in rats. *Neuroimage* 2011;54 Suppl 1:S89–97.

83. I. Cernak. The importance of systemic response in the pathobiology of blast-induced neurotrauma. *Front Neurol* 2010;1:151.

84. A. Kamnaksh, E. Kovesdi, S.K. Kwon, et al. Factors affecting blast traumatic brain injury. *J Neurotrauma* 2011;28 (10):2145–53.

85. D.V. Agoston, A. Gyorgy, O. Eidelman, H.B. Pollard. Proteomic biomarkers for blast neurotrauma: targeting cerebral edema, inflammation, and neuronal death cascades. *J Neurotrauma* 2009;26 (6):901–11.

86. G.A. Elder, N.P. Dorr, R. De Gasperi, et al. Blast exposure induces post-traumatic stress disorder-related traits in a rat model of mild traumatic brain injury. *J Neurotrauma* 2012;29(16):2564–75.

87. E. Kovesdi, A. Kamnaksh, D. Wingo, et al. Acute minocycline treatment mitigates the symptoms of mild blast-induced traumatic brain injury. *Front Neurol* 2012;3:111.

88. S.K. Kwon, E. Kovesdi, A.B. Gyorgy, et al. Stress and traumatic brain injury: a behavioral, proteomics, and histological study. *Front Neurol* 2011;2:12.

89. A. Kamnaksh, S.K. Kwon, E. Kovesdi, et al. Neurobehavioral, cellular, and molecular consequences of single and multiple mild blast exposure. *Electrophoresis* 2012;33 (24):3680–92.

90. V. Bugay, E. Bozdemir, F.A. Vigil, et al. A mouse model of repetitive blast traumatic brain injury reveals post-trauma seizures and increased neuronal excitability. *J Neurotrauma* 2020;37(2):248–61.

91. X.C. Lu, J.A. Hartings, Y. Si, A. Balbir, Y. Cao, F.C. Tortella. Electrocortical pathology in a rat model of penetrating ballistic-like brain injury. *J Neurotrauma* 2011;28(1):71–83.

92. D.A. Shear, X.C. Lu, M.C. Bombard, et al. Longitudinal characterization of motor and cognitive deficits in a model of penetrating ballistic-like brain injury. *J Neurotrauma* 2010;27(10):1911–23.

93. A.J. Williams, J.A. Hartings, X.C. Lu, M.L. Rolli, J.R. Dave, F.C. Tortella. Characterization of a new rat model of penetrating ballistic brain injury. *J Neurotrauma* 2005;22(2):313–31.

94. M.T. Kendirli, D.T. Rose, E.H. Bertram. A model of posttraumatic epilepsy after penetrating brain injuries: effect of lesion size and metal fragments. *Epilepsia* 2014;55 (12):1969–77.

95. D.M. Feeney, M.G. Boyeson, R.T. Linn, H.M. Murray, W.G. Dail. Responses to cortical injury: I. Methodology and local effects of contusions in the rat. *Brain Res* 1981;211(1):67–77.

96. W.G. Dail, D.M. Feeney, H.M. Murray, R.T. Linn, M.G. Boyeson. Responses to cortical injury: II. Widespread depression of the activity of an enzyme in cortex remote from a focal injury. *Brain Res* 1981;211(1):79–89.

97. C. Gasparovic, N. Arfai, N. Smid, D.M. Feeney. Decrease and recovery of N-acetylaspartate/creatine in rat brain remote from focal injury. *J Neurotrauma* 2001;18(3):241–6.

98. A. Marmarou, M.A. Foda, W. van den Brink, J. Campbell, H. Kita, K. Demetriadou. A new model of diffuse brain injury in rats. Part I: Pathophysiology and biomechanics. *J Neurosurg* 1994;80(2):291–300.

99. D.L. Heath, R. Vink. Impact acceleration-induced severe diffuse axonal injury in rats: characterization of phosphate metabolism and neurologic outcome. *J Neurotrauma* 1995;12 (6):1027–34.

100. R.H. Schmidt, K.J. Scholten, P.H. Maughan. Cognitive impairment and synaptosomal choline uptake in rats following impact acceleration injury. *J Neurotrauma* 2000;17(12):1129–39.

101. M.A. Foda, A. Marmarou. A new model of diffuse brain injury in rats. Part II: Morphological characterization. *J Neurosurg* 1994;80(2):301–13.

102. M.A. Flierl, P.F. Stahel, K.M. Beauchamp, S.J. Morgan, W.R. Smith, E. Shohami. Mouse closed head injury model induced by a weight-drop device. *Nat Protoc.* 2009;4(9):1328–37.

103. Y. Chen, S. Constantini, V. Trembovler, M. Weinstock, E. Shohami. An experimental model of closed head injury in mice: pathophysiology, histopathology, and cognitive deficits. *J Neurotrauma* 1996;13(10):557–68.

104. C. Albert-Weissenberger, C. Varrallyay, F. Raslan, C. Kleinschnitz, A.L. Siren. An experimental protocol for mimicking pathomechanisms of traumatic brain injury in mice. *Exp Transl Stroke Med* 2012;4:1.

105. P.D. Adelson, C.E. Dixon, P.M. Kochanek. Long-term dysfunction following diffuse traumatic brain injury in the immature rat. *J Neurotrauma* 2000;17 (4):273–82.

106. P.D. Adelson, M.J. Whalen, P.M. Kochanek, P. Robichaud, T.M. Carlos. Blood brain barrier permeability and acute inflammation in two models of traumatic brain injury in the immature rat: a preliminary report. *Acta Neurochir Suppl* 1998;71:104–6.

107. J.W. Huh, A.G. Widing, R. Raghupathi. Midline brain injury in the immature rat induces sustained cognitive deficits, bihemispheric axonal injury and neurodegeneration. *Exp Neurol* 2008;213 (1):84–92.

108. P.D. Adelson, L.W. Jenkins, R.L. Hamilton, P. Robichaud, M.P. Tran, P.M. Kochanek. Histopathologic response of the immature rat to diffuse traumatic brain injury. *J Neurotrauma* 2001;18 (10):967–76.

109. P.D. Adelson, W. Fellows-Mayle, P.M. Kochanek, C.E. Dixon. Morris water maze function and histologic characterization of two age-at-injury experimental models of controlled cortical impact in the immature rat. *Childs Nerv Sys* 2013;29(1):43–53.

110. S.G. Kernie, J.M. Parent. Forebrain neurogenesis after focal ischemic and traumatic brain injury. *Neurobiol Dis* 2010;37(2):267–74.

111. D. Sun, R.J. Colello, W.P. Daugherty, et al. Cell proliferation and neuronal differentiation in the dentate gyrus in juvenile and adult rats following traumatic brain injury. *J Neurotrauma* 2005;22(1):95–105.

112. M.T. Goodus, A.M. Guzman, F. Calderon, Y. Jiang, S.W. Levison. Neural stem cells in the immature, but not the mature, subventricular zone respond robustly to traumatic brain injury. *Develop Neurosci* 2015;37(1):29–42.

113. E.J. Neuberger, B. Swietek, L. Corrubia, A. Prasanna, V. Santhakumar. Enhanced dentate neurogenesis after brain injury undermines long-term neurogenic potential and promotes seizure susceptibility. *Stem Cell Rep* 2017;9 (3):972–84.

114. S.W. Scheff, D.A. Price, R.R. Hicks, S.A. Baldwin, S. Robinson, C. Brackney. Synaptogenesis in the hippocampal CA1 field following traumatic brain injury. *J Neurotrauma* 2005;22(7):719–32.

115. E.M. Casella, T.C. Thomas, D.L. Vanino, et al. Traumatic brain injury alters long-term hippocampal neuron

morphology in juvenile, but not immature, rats. *Childs Nerv Sys* 2014;30 (8):1333–42.

116. R. Mychasiuk, A. Farran, M.J. Esser. Assessment of an experimental rodent model of pediatric mild traumatic brain injury. *J Neurotrauma* 2014;31 (8):749–57.

117. J. Nichols, R. Perez, C. Wu, P.D. Adelson, T. Anderson. Traumatic brain injury induces rapid enhancement of cortical excitability in juvenile rats. *CNS Neurosci Ther* 2015;21(2):193–203.

118. S.W. Scheff, L.S. Benardo, C.W. Cotman. Decline in reactive fiber growth in the dentate gyrus of aged rats compared to young adult rats following entorhinal cortex removal. *Brain Res* 1980;199 (1):21–38.

119. N. Li, Y. Yang, D.P. Glover, et al. Evidence for impaired plasticity after traumatic brain injury in the developing brain. *J Neurotrauma* 2014;31(4):395–403.

120. M.B. Potts, S.E. Koh, W.D. Whetstone, et al. Traumatic injury to the immature brain: inflammation, oxidative injury, and iron-mediated damage as potential therapeutic targets. *NeuroRx* 2006;3 (2):143–53.

121. T. Ravizza, A. Vezzani. Pharmacological targeting of brain inflammation in epilepsy: Therapeutic perspectives from experimental and clinical studies. *Epilepsia Open* 2018;3 (Suppl 2):133–42.

122. C.P. Claus, K. Tsuru-Aoyagi, H. Adwanikar, B. Walker, W. Whetstone, L.J. Noble-Haeusslein. Age is a determinant of leukocyte infiltration and loss of cortical volume after traumatic brain injury. *Develop Neurosci* 2010;32(5–6):454–65.

123. J.Y. Khan, S.M. Black. Developmental changes in murine brain antioxidant enzymes. *Pediatr Res* 2003;54(1):77–82.

124. A. Aspberg, O. Tottmar. Development of antioxidant enzymes in rat brain and in reaggregation culture of fetal brain cells. *Brain Res Develop Brain Res* 1992;66 (1):55–8.

125. A. Buard, M. Clement, J.M. Bourre. Developmental changes in enzymatic systems involved in protection against peroxidation in isolated rat brain microvessels. *Neurosci Lett* 1992;141 (1):72–4.

126. O. Lazo, A.K. Singh, I. Singh. Postnatal development and isolation of peroxisomes from brain. *J Neurochem* 1991;56(4):1343–53.

127. B.A. Holshouser, S. Ashwal, G.Y. Luh, et al. Proton MR spectroscopy after acute central nervous system injury: outcome prediction in neonates, infants, and children. *Radiology* 1997;202(2):487–96.

128. S. Ashwal, B.A. Holshouser, S.K. Shu, et al. Predictive value of proton magnetic resonance spectroscopy in pediatric closed head injury. *Pediatr Neurol* 2000;23 (2):114–25.

129. S. Scafidi, J. O'Brien, I. Hopkins, C. Robertson, G. Fiskum, M. McKenna. Delayed cerebral oxidative glucose metabolism after traumatic brain injury in young rats. *J Neurochem* 2009;109 Suppl 1:189–97.

130. P.A. Casey, M.C. McKenna, G. Fiskum, M. Saraswati, C.L. Robertson. Early and sustained alterations in cerebral metabolism after traumatic brain injury in immature rats. *J Neurotrauma* 2008;25 (6):603–14.

131. C.L. Robertson, M. Saraswati, S. Scafidi, G. Fiskum, P. Casey, M.C. McKenna. Cerebral glucose metabolism in an immature rat model of pediatric traumatic brain injury. *J Neurotrauma* 2013;30(24):2066–72.

132. Y. Deng-Bryant, M.L. Prins, D.A. Hovda, N.G. Harris. Ketogenic diet prevents alterations in brain metabolism in young but not adult rats after traumatic brain injury. *J Neurotrauma* 2011;28 (9):1813–25.

133. M.L. Prins, J. Matsumoto. Metabolic response of pediatric traumatic brain injury. *J Child Neurol* 2016;31(1):28–34.

134. P.A. Schwartzkroin, H.J. Wenzel, B.G. Lyeth, et al. Does ketogenic diet alter seizure sensitivity and cell loss following

fluid percussion injury? *Epilepsy Res* 2010;92(1):74–84.

135. A.S. Galanopoulou, J.A. Gorter, C. Cepeda. Finding a better drug for epilepsy: the mTOR pathway as an antiepileptogenic target. *Epilepsia* 2012;53 (7):1119–30.

136. C.R. Butler, J.A. Boychuk, B.N. Smith. Effects of rapamycin treatment on neurogenesis and synaptic reorganization in the dentate gyrus after controlled cortical impact injury in mice. *Front Syst Neurosci* 2015;9:163.

137. C. Wang, Z. Hu, Y. Zou, et al. The post-therapeutic effect of rapamycin in mild traumatic brain-injured rats ensuing in the upregulation of autophagy and mitophagy. *Cell Biol Int* 2017;41 (9):1039–47.

138. L.J. Willmore, R.W. Hurd, G.W. Sypert. Epileptiform activity initiated by pial iontophoresis of ferrous and ferric chloride on rat cerebral cortex. *Brain Res* 1978;152(2):406–10.

139. E. Ronne Engstrom, L. Hillered, R. Flink, et al. Extracellular amino acid levels measured with intracerebral microdialysis in the model of posttraumatic epilepsy induced by intracortical iron injection. *Epilepsy Res* 2001;43(2):135–44.

140. P.G. Saletti, C.P. Lisgaras, P. Casillas-Espinosa, et al. (eds.) Site and time-specific tau hyperphosphorylation patterns in the rat cerebral cortex after traumatic brain injury: An EpiBioS4Rx Project 2 study. *Society for Neuroscience Annual Meeting*; 2019; Chicago, IL: Society for Neuroscience.

141. P.M. Kochanek, H.M. Bramlett, C.E. Dixon, et al. Operation brain trauma therapy: 2016 update. *Mil Med* 2018;183 (suppl_1):303–12.

142. A.S. Galanopoulou, J. Engel, Jr., S.L. Moshe. Preface: Antiepileptogenesis following traumatic brain injury. *Neurobiol Dis* 2019;123:1–2.

143. J. Engel, Jr. Epileptogenesis, traumatic brain injury, and biomarkers. *Neurobiol Dis* 2019;123:3–7.

144. C.E. Dixon, B.G. Lyeth, J.T. Povlishock, et al. A fluid percussion model of experimental brain injury in the rat. *J Neurosurg* 1987;67(1):110–9.

145. R. D'Ambrosio, S. Hakimian, T. Stewart, et al. Functional definition of seizure provides new insight into post-traumatic epileptogenesis. *Brain* 2009;132 (10):2805–21.

146. C.C. Giza, M.L. Prins, D.A. Hovda, H.R. Herschman, J.D. Feldman. Genes preferentially induced by depolarization after concussive brain injury: effects of age and injury severity. *J Neurotrauma* 2002;19(4):387–402.

147. E.Y. Ip, C.C. Giza, G.S. Griesbach, D.A. Hovda. Effects of enriched environment and fluid percussion injury on dendritic arborization within the cerebral cortex of the developing rat. *J Neurotrauma* 2002;19(5):573–85.

148. G.S. Griesbach, D.A. Hovda, R. Molteni, F. Gomez-Pinilla. Alterations in BDNF and synapsin I within the occipital cortex and hippocampus after mild traumatic brain injury in the developing rat: reflections of injury-induced neuroplasticity. *J Neurotrauma* 2002;19 (7):803–14.

149. P.B. de la Tremblaye, C.O. Bondi, N. Lajud, J.P. Cheng, H.L. Radabaugh, A.E. Kline. Galantamine and environmental enrichment enhance cognitive recovery after experimental traumatic brain injury but do not confer additional benefits when combined. *J Neurotrauma* 2017;34(8):1610–22.

150. N.K. Liu, Y.P. Zhang, J. Zou, et al. A semicircular controlled cortical impact produces long-term motor and cognitive dysfunction that correlates well with damage to both the sensorimotor cortex and hippocampus. *Brain Res* 2014;1576:18–26.

151. M.J. Hylin, R.C. Holden, A.C. Smith, A.F. Logsdon, R. Qaiser, B.P. Lucke-Wold. Juvenile traumatic brain injury results in cognitive deficits associated with impaired endoplasmic reticulum stress and early tauopathy. *Develop Neurosci* 2018;40(2):175–88.

152. B.D. Semple, A. Trivedi, K. Gimlin, L. J. Noble-Haeusslein. Neutrophil elastase mediates acute pathogenesis and is a determinant of long-term behavioral recovery after traumatic injury to the immature brain. *Neurobiol Dis* 2015;74:263–80.

153. S.W. Lee, M.S. Jang, S.H. Jeong, H. Kim. Exploratory, cognitive, and depressive-like behaviors in adult and pediatric mice exposed to controlled cortical impact. *Clin Exp Emerg Med* 2019;6(2):125–37.

154. J. Nissinen, P. Andrade, T. Natunen, et al. Disease-modifying effect of atipamezole in a model of post-traumatic epilepsy. *Epilepsy Res* 2017;136:18–34.

155. G.S. Goodrich, A.Y. Kabakov, M.Q. Hameed, S.C. Dhamne, P.A. Rosenberg, A. Rotenberg. Ceftriaxone treatment after traumatic brain injury restores expression of the glutamate transporter, GLT-1, reduces regional gliosis, and reduces post-traumatic seizures in the rat. *J Neurotrauma* 2013;30(16):1434–41.

156. R. D'Ambrosio, C.L. Eastman, F. Darvas, et al. Mild passive focal cooling prevents epileptic seizures after head injury in rats. *Ann Neurol* 2013;73(2):199–209.

Chapter 2

Post-traumatic Epilepsy: Epidemiology, Definition and Terminology

Peter Jenkins and Hannah Cock

Introduction

Epileptic seizures are common following a traumatic brain injury (TBI)[1] and are associated with a worse clinical outcome.[2, 3] They frequently occur at the time of an injury (or very soon after) due to an acute disruption to normal brain structure and physiology, but they can also develop many years later.[1] Early seizures (defined as those occurring within a week of injury) are not an independent risk factor for the development of future seizures,[1] whereas the risk of further seizures after a single late post-traumatic seizure (occurring more than a week after injury) can be as high as 80%.[4]

TBI is very common, with an estimated 50 million people worldwide suffering a TBI each year.[5] Given its high prevalence and its risk for the development of epilepsy, TBI is a major cause of acquired epilepsy, with population-based studies estimating it to be the basis of around 6% of all cases of epilepsy.[6]

Epilepsy, more properly termed 'the epilepsies' encompassing hundreds of different types and causes, similarly affects over 50 million people worldwide.[7] Up to 5% of people will have a seizure at some point in their life,[8] with an estimated 1 in 26 people developing epilepsy during their lifetime.[9] An epileptic seizure is defined as a transient occurrence of signs and/or symptoms due to abnormal excessive or synchronous neuronal activity in the brain. Having seizures does not, however, constitute a diagnosis of epilepsy. Almost any brain might generate a seizure at the time of a sufficiently severe insult (e.g. metabolic, toxic, inflammatory or traumatic), and this is termed an acute symptomatic or provoked seizure.[10] The risk of recurrence after acute symptomatic seizures is low (1–3%), other than in individuals repeatedly exposed to the same trigger (e.g. alcohol withdrawal). Epilepsy is defined as the enduring predisposition to generate unprovoked epileptic seizures.[11] From a practical perspective, the occurrence of two unprovoked seizures more than 24 hours apart has long been recognized to indicate a diagnosis of epilepsy as the risk of further seizures is high (60–90%) in this context.[12] However, as we shall go on to discuss, it is now accepted that if other evidence supports a high (>60%) probability of recurrent seizures occurring after one seizure, a diagnosis of epilepsy should be made rather than waiting for a second seizure to occur. Evidence of increased risk of future seizures includes epileptic abnormalities on EEG, structural changes on brain imaging known to be highly predictive of increased risk and epidemiological evidence in relation to individual aetiologies. The risk of a recurrent seizure after a first unprovoked event in an individual can vary from <10% to >90% depending on these and other variables.[13] Traumatic brain injury can precipitate acute symptomatic seizures but can also cause long-lasting structural and physiological changes in the brain that can predispose to epileptic seizures. Understanding the risks of seizures and accurately diagnosing epilepsy after a TBI is important to facilitate counselling and aid treatment decisions whilst avoiding unnecessary medication use.

To support clinical decision-making, several large epidemiological studies have attempted to quantify the risks of seizures after TBI. In this chapter, we outline and summarize the results from the largest studies. These studies have provided valuable information on the incidence of post-traumatic epilepsy (PTE). In particular, they highlight the significant increased risk of epilepsy conferred by a TBI and show, perhaps surprisingly, that this risk persists for many years after the injury (over 20 years for a severe TBI[1]). Severity of injury, presence of intracranial haemorrhage, length of post-traumatic amnesia, length of loss of consciousness and time after injury are all clear predictors of seizure risk. In addition, other factors, including the presence of additional medical comorbidities, depression and a family history of epilepsy, may also increase the risk of the development of PTE.[14, 15] These factors highlight that the development of epilepsy is likely to be a multifactorial process, dependent on the characteristics of the individual as well as the injury itself.

Definitions and Terminology for Post-traumatic Epilepsy

In order to understand the potential risks of PTE and the relationship to TBI severity, it is important to appreciate how epilepsy, PTE and TBI severity are defined and classified.

A Practical Definition for Epilepsy

The current conceptual definitions of epilepsy and epileptic seizures were formulated in 2005 by the International League Against Epilepsy (ILAE)[16]:

> *Epileptic seizure:* A transient occurrence of signs and/or symptoms due to abnormal excessive or synchronous neuronal activity in the brain.
> *Epilepsy:* A disorder of the brain characterized by an enduring predisposition to generate epileptic seizures, and by the neurobiological, psychological and social consequences of this condition. The definition of epilepsy requires the occurrence of at least one epileptic seizure.

At the time these definitions were proposed, the diagnosis of epilepsy required the occurrence of two unprovoked seizures at least 24 hours apart. The rationale for this requirement was based on epidemiological data showing the risk of recurrence after a single unprovoked seizure is 30–50%.[17] Following a second unprovoked seizure, this risk rises to 60–90%.[12] Exposing an individual to the potential harm of treatment therefore seems reasonable after two but probably not one seizure. However, despite the value of this working definition, it became increasingly apparent that it was inadequate in certain situations. In particular, it did not address situations where there was a high risk of future seizures after a single unprovoked seizure. For example, individuals who have suffered a remote brain insult (e.g. stroke or traumatic injury) have a comparable risk of a second unprovoked seizure to those suffering two unprovoked seizures.[18]

This is now articulated in the practical, operational clinical definition of epilepsy put forward in 2014,[11] which states:

> Epilepsy is a disease of the brain defined by any of the following conditions:
> 1. At least two unprovoked (or reflex) seizures occurring >24 h apart

2. One unprovoked (or reflex) seizure and a probability of further seizures similar to the general recurrence risk (at least 60%) after two unprovoked seizures, occurring over the next 10 years
3. Diagnosis of an epilepsy syndrome

Epilepsy is considered to be resolved for individuals who had an age-dependent epilepsy syndrome but are now past the applicable age or those who have remained seizure-free for the last 10 years, with no seizure medicines for the last 5 years.

This update in the working definition is important as the treatment goal in the management of epilepsy is reducing the mortality and morbidity associated with seizures. Therefore, it is logical that the decision to initiate treatment should be based on future risk of seizures rather than necessarily waiting for a second seizure to occur. It is difficult to provide a specific risk threshold at which an individual is considered to have 'epilepsy' rather than an isolated unprovoked seizure, but it seems reasonable to assume that an individual with a predisposition for further seizures comparable to that following two unprovoked seizures should also be considered to have epilepsy and managed as such.

The classification and terminology relating to seizures[19] and epilepsies[20] were also updated in 2017. Previous classification systems, particularly in relation to focal onset (previously termed partial) seizures, did not adequately capture the range of different seizure types. In addition, some felt the term 'partial' inferred these were less important or incomplete seizures/epilepsies, whereas in reality they are often the most disabling and difficult to control. Currently recommended terms and mapping to prior terminology is summarized in Table 2.1.

The new classification comprises three levels of classification and six aetiological groups as summarized in Figure 2.1. The starting point of this framework is to define the seizure onset as focal, generalized or unknown. The second level is epilepsy type, including focal, generalized, combined generalized and focal and unknown. Some individuals may have both.

Table 2.1 Summary of common terminology for types of seizures used by lay people and how this maps to the previous and current classification

Lay term	Previous terminology	Current terminology (ILAE 2017)
Convulsion, Grand Mal, seizure	Generalized tonic-clonic seizure, secondary generalized tonic-clonic seizure	Generalized tonic-clonic seizure focal to bilateral tonic-clonic seizure
Absence, blank, petit mal	Complex partial seizure Absence seizure	Focal impaired awareness absence seizure
Funnies, turns, déjà vu, aura, warning, partial, small seizure	Partial seizures (multiple types)	Focal seizures (multiple types)
Drop attack	Atonic seizure, tonic seizure, partial seizure	Atonic seizure, tonic seizure, focal seizure, nonepileptic
Jerk, twitch	Myoclonic seizure, simple partial seizure	Myoclonic seizure, focal motor seizure.

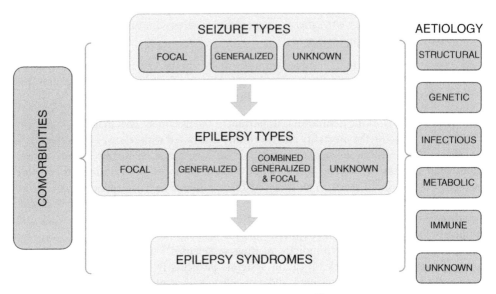

Figure 2.1 Framework of ILAE classification of the epilepsies 2017, from.[20]

For example, a patient with a generalized epilepsy syndrome, such as juvenile myoclonic epilepsy, may also suffer a TBI and acquire post-traumatic focal epilepsy. The third level is of an epilepsy syndrome diagnosis where one exists. An epilepsy syndrome refers to a collection of qualities including seizure type, EEG and imaging features. Typical examples of well-recognized epilepsy syndromes include Dravet syndrome and childhood absence epilepsy.

Any diagnosis of epilepsy should also include the cause where possible and identification of any important comorbidities. For most individuals, the appropriate category will either be obvious or unknown. However, some will seem to straddle more than one group. For example, tuberous sclerosis is a known genetic condition, yet would be classified as a structural cause, as the 'dominant' contributor to the risk of seizures is the associated structural brain abnormality. By definition, PTE would involve focal onset seizures and be considered structural in terms of aetiology, even though there may be metabolic factors involved in triggering seizures and the development of epilepsy.

Post-traumatic Seizures and Post-traumatic Epilepsy

Seizures following trauma are classified based on their timing in relation to the injury, as this has important prognostic implications with regards to the risk of future seizures. The presence of seizures occurring within the first 7 days after a TBI is a strong risk factor for late seizures. However, this increased risk is almost entirely eliminated with adjustment for other prognostic factors such as injury severity.[1] Early seizures of themselves do not confer a sufficiently high risk of subsequent recurrent seizures to warrant long-term treatment and a diagnosis of epilepsy. They are therefore considered acute symptomatic seizures. In contrast, even a single late seizure (>7 days after injury) does confer a substantial risk of future unprovoked seizures, that is, the development of PTE.[18]

A large epidemiological study illustrating this analysed the prognosis after a first acute symptomatic seizure (occurring within 7 days of the TBI) and after a first unprovoked seizure (>7 days after injury) in terms of short- and long-term mortality and risk of subsequent unprovoked seizures.[18] Individuals with a first acute symptomatic seizure compared with a first unprovoked seizure were significantly more likely to die within the first 30 days after the seizure (11%, 95% CI (6.1–19.6%) vs. 0%) and less likely to experience a subsequent unprovoked seizure over the next 10 years (13.4% (95% CI=7.0–24.8%) vs. 46.6% (95% CI=30.4–66.3%)). There was no difference in mortality at 10 years between the two groups. From this analysis the authors concluded that early and late seizures following a TBI are different entities with different prognoses. Furthermore, early seizures are not associated with an 'enduring predisposition to generate epileptic seizures' and should therefore not be considered as a marker for the development of epilepsy.

Classification of Traumatic Brain Injury Severity

As detailed in the following section, different epidemiological studies employed different definitions for TBI severity. There is a clear link between TBI severity and risk of development of PTE, although there is no uniform consensus on how severity should be defined. A combination of length of post-traumatic amnesia, length of loss of consciousness, Glasgow Coma Score, presence of skull fracture and presence of structural brain injury (e.g. contusion, cerebral or extra-cerebral haematoma) are the most commonly used indicators. Differentiating between penetrating and nonpenetrating TBI is also important, as the risk of PTE after a penetrating injury is far higher (case series report around 50% risk of PTE in military personnel suffering penetrating head injuries[21]).

Additionally, neuroimaging has only become commonplace over the last 30–40 years and therefore the older epidemiological studies do not include it in their assessment of severity. However, neuroimaging is an important indicator of TBI severity[22] and therefore a key component in more recent TBI severity classifications (e.g. the Mayo classification for TBI severity[23]).

The TBI severity classification systems used in the epidemiological studies include the head Abbreviated Injury Scale (AIS), the International Classification of Diseases (ICD) and combined clinical markers, including the Glasgow Coma Scale (GCS), length of post-traumatic amnesia, length of loss of consciousness, skull fracture, subdural haematoma, brain contusion or intracerebral haemorrhage. The GCS is commonly used to stratify severity of TBI, with a score of 13–15 considered mild, 9–12 moderate and 3–8 severe.[24] However, its use can be confounded by other factors not attributable to the TBI, such as length of time between injury and assessment, early sedation and extra-cranial injuries. In addition, individuals with structural injuries present on neuroimaging but GCS 13 or greater have been shown to have outcomes more consistent with a moderate rather than mild injury, suggesting GCS alone can underestimate severity.[22] The head AIS ranks anatomic injury on a scale of 1 (least severe) to 6 (most severe).[25] It uses standardized terminology to stratify the severity of injury and has been shown to weakly correlate with functional outcome.[26–28] Finally, the ICD has been used in some epidemiological studies to classify TBI severity.[29, 30] These studies used the following ICD codes for stratification: ICD-9-CM 850 = Mild, ICD-9-CM 851–854 = Severe and ICD-9-CM 800–804 to signify the presence of a skull fracture. Mild TBI is classified as 'concussion' (ICD-9-CM 850) with or without loss of consciousness that can be greater than 24 hours and without a return to pre-existing conscious level. There is no consensus agreement on what constitutes a diagnosis of concussion,[31] making its use problematic in classifying injury severity. In addition, most clinicians would consider a head injury with loss of consciousness greater than 24 hours and without a return to pre-existing conscious level (even without intracerebral haemorrhage or skull fracture) to be a severe brain injury. The severe TBI classification only includes patients with evidence of cerebral contusion, traumatic subarachnoid haemorrhage, extradural haemorrhage or subdural haemorrhage.

Epidemiology of Post-traumatic Epilepsy

The risk of developing PTE is dependent on injury severity and type, ranging from 2% after mild injuries to over 50% following penetrating injuries.[1, 15, 21] Given the high incidence of TBI, with around 50 million people worldwide suffering a TBI each year,[5] the prevalence of PTE is also very high. In addition, the prevalence of TBI as the causative factor for epilepsy varies by age group due to the varying incidence of TBI and other factors influencing risk of epilepsy (e.g. stroke) in different age groups. In one study, nearly 30% of epilepsy cases where a cause could be determined were attributed to a TBI in the 15–34-year-old age group, whereas it only accounted for 14% in younger children and 8% in adults over the age of 65 years given the increasing likelihood of other factors in this group (e.g. stroke).[6]

The risk of early seizures (within the first 7 days of injury) varies between 2% and 17% and is dependent on injury severity and age.[32] In isolation, early seizures are a strong risk factor for the development of late seizures; however, when other factors such as injury severity are taken into account this risk is removed. Hence, early seizures do not appear to be an independent risk factor for the development of PTE.[1] Seizures can develop many years after a TBI, with an enduring risk above that of the matched population even 20 years after a severe TBI.[1] The risk of seizure recurrence after a single late seizure (>1 week after injury) is high (over 80%[4]) and therefore these individuals need counselling regarding future seizure risk and anti-epileptic treatment to reduce the risk of further seizures.

Evidence for Post-traumatic Seizure Risk

Several large epidemiological studies have attempted to determine the effect of TBI on the future risk of seizures. The results of the largest studies are summarized in Table 2.2. Due to methodological differences, it is not possible to pool the data from all studies and specific limitations for each study need to be borne in mind. In particular, not all studies use a comparison group, which given the incidence of seizures in the general population is a significant flaw. In addition, the utility of retrospective studies is dependent on the validity of the diagnoses and the generalizability of the results from the population studied. Finally, given the evidence that the risk of PTE can persist for over 30 years after the injury, the length of follow-up is an important factor and a major reason why it is difficult to conduct these studies.

Annegers et al. conducted a large retrospective population-based case-control study that identified 4,541 children and adults of all ages who suffered a TBI between 1935 and 1984 in a US county using medical records.[1] The chance of developing epilepsy in these patients was compared with that of the age-matched population, giving an estimate of the risk associated with TBI. They categorized the brain injury into mild (loss of consciousness or amnesia lasting less than 30 minutes), moderate (loss of consciousness or amnesia for 30 minutes to 24 hours or a skull fracture) and severe (loss of consciousness or amnesia for more than 24 hours, subdural haematoma or brain contusion). As computed tomography (CT) imaging

Table 2.2 Largest studies investigating risk of seizures after traumatic brain injury

Study	Study design	No. of individuals suffering a TBI	TBI categorization criteria	Number of people suffering unprovoked seizures	Increased likelihood of developing seizures	Predictors of future seizure risk
Annegers et al. 1998[1]	Retrospective population-based case–control study. All ages.	4,541	Mild: Loss of consciousness or amnesia <30 minutes	97	1.5 times	Brain contusion, subdural haematoma, depressed skull fracture, loss of consciousness or post-traumatic amnesia >24 hours
			Moderate: Loss of consciousness or amnesia >30 minutes or skull fracture		2.9 times	
			Severe: Loss of consciousness or amnesia >24 hours, subdural haematoma or contusion		17 times	
Christensen et al. 2009[15]	Retrospective population-based case–control study on people born in	78,572	Skull fracture	1,017	2.2 times	Severity of injury, age at time of injury, female gender, family history of epilepsy

Table 2.2 (cont.)

Study	Study design	No. of individuals suffering a TBI	TBI categorization criteria	Number of people suffering unprovoked seizures	Increased likelihood of developing seizures	Predictors of future seizure risk
	Denmark between 1977 and 2002					
	Children and young adults.		Mild: Relevant trauma to the head and loss of consciousness (<30 minutes), amnesia (<24 hours), confusion or focal, temporary neurological deficit. GCS >13 after 30 minutes		2.2 times	
			Severe: Evidence of structural brain injury (e.g. contusion or intracranial haemorrhage)		7.4 times	
Ferguson et al. 2010[14]	Prospective follow up study. Individuals aged ≥15 years.	2,118 (followed up at 1 year) 1,165	Mild: AIS=2	115	4.4 cases of PTE per 100 persons over 3 years[b]	Severe TBI, multiple chronic medical conditions, history of depression, history of post-

Followed up for 4 years.	(followed-up at 3 years)		traumatic seizures prior to hospital discharge
	Loss of consciousness <15 minutes, linear skull fracture		
	Moderate: AIS=3	7.6 cases of PTE per 100 persons over 3 years[b]	
	Loss of consciousness 15–59 minutes, depressed or base of skull fracture with no CSF leak, subarachnoid haemorrhage or brain contusion		
	Severe: AIS=4,5	13.6 cases of PTE per 100 persons over 3 years[b]	
	Loss of consciousness greater than 1 hour, subdural haemorrhage, fracture of base of skull with CSF leak		

Table 2.2 (cont.)

Study	Study design	No. of individuals suffering a TBI	TBI categorization criteria	Number of people suffering unprovoked seizures	Increased likelihood of developing seizures	Predictors of future seizure risk
Zhao et al. 2012[34]	Retrospective population-based study on patients discharged from a brain trauma centre in China between 2004 and 2008. No control group. All ages.	2,826	Mild: GCS on admission to hospital of 13–15	141	3.6%[b]	Age, severity of injury, skull fracture, abnormal brain imaging, presence of early seizures
			Moderate: GCS on admission to hospital of 9–12		6.9%[b]	
			Severe: GCS on admission to hospital of 3–8		17[b]	
Yeh et al. 2013[30]	Retrospective population-based case-control study based on national registry. Individuals aged ≥ 15 years.	19,336	Mild: ICD-9-CM 850: Concussion[a] with or without loss of consciousness	1,553	3.0 times higher	Male gender, age at time of injury, severity of injury
			Severe: ICD-9-CM 851–854: Cerebral contusion, traumatic subarachnoid		5.1 times higher	

	5–8 year follow-up period.		haemorrhage, extradural haemorrhage or subdural haemorrhage		
			Skull fracture: ICD-9-CM 800–804: Fracture of skull vault or base of skull	10.6 times higher	Intracerebral haemorrhage, contusion
Mahler et al. 2015[29]	Retrospective population-based case-control study based on an epilepsy registry and subsequent identification of prior TBI. All ages.	105 (number of patients with an unprovoked seizure and prior TBI)	Mild: ICD-9-CM 850: Concussion[a] with or without loss of consciousness	1,885	
			Severe: ICD-9-CM 851–854: Cerebral contusion, traumatic subarachnoid haemorrhage, extradural haemorrhage or subdural haemorrhage	2.0 times higher	

Table 2.2 (cont.)

Study	Study design	No. of individuals suffering a TBI	TBI categorization criteria	Number of people suffering unprovoked seizures	Increased likelihood of developing seizures	Predictors of future seizure risk
			Skull fracture: ICD-9-CM 800–803: Fracture of skull vault or base of skull		8.1 times higher	
					4.5 times higher	

[a] See text regarding diagnosis of concussion.
[b] No control group for relative risk.
PTE, Post-traumatic epilepsy; ICD, International Classification of Diseases; AIS, Abbreviated Injury Scale; GCS, Glasgow Coma Score.

was only available for the final 10 years of the study, contusions were diagnosed on the basis of observation during surgery or on the presence of focal neurologic symptoms.

In total, 97 patients suffered unprovoked seizures during the follow-up period, which ranged from days to decades. Of these, 22 had just one seizure and 75 had multiple seizures. The severity of the injury affected both the overall risk of epilepsy and the length of period at risk. Patients suffering a severe TBI were 17 times more likely to develop epilepsy than matched controls, those with a moderate TBI were 2.9 times more likely and mild TBI conferred a 1.5 times increased risk. Approximately half of the people who were going to develop epilepsy did so within 1 year of the TBI and three-quarters within 5 years. The length of period at risk was also related to the severity of the injury, with an increased risk of seizures persisting for 5, 10 and >20 years for mild, moderate and severe injuries respectively.

The strongest predictors of future seizure risk were the presence of a brain contusion or subdural haematoma. In addition, depressed skull fractures and loss of consciousness or post-traumatic amnesia lasting longer than 24 hours were independent predictors of future seizure risk. The presence of early seizures was not an independent predictor of future risk of late seizures. This was the first large population based study giving information on the risk of development of PTE. The main limitations of this study include the reliance on medical records that may not be complete or accurate, a high dropout rate of 25% and importantly modern neuroimaging was not available for the majority of patients.

Christensen et al. conducted a large population-based case-control study on more than 1.6 million children and young adults born in Denmark between 1977 and 2002.[15] Patients were classified as suffering a skull fracture or mild or severe TBI. Mild TBI was defined as a history of a relevant trauma to the head with altered brain function (i.e. loss of conscious-ness, amnesia, confusion or focal, temporary neurological deficit). Loss of consciousness had to be less than 30 minutes, post-traumatic amnesia less than 24 hours and Glasgow Coma Score (GCS) 13 or greater after 30 minutes. A severe TBI was defined as evidence of a structural brain injury (e.g. contusion or intracranial haemorrhage).

Over 78,000 individuals were identified as suffering a TBI in this study. The subse-quent risk of epilepsy was 2.2 times higher after a mild TBI, 7.4 times higher after a severe TBI and 2.2 times higher after a skull fracture. The rate of development of epilepsy was greatest in the few years after the head injury with a greater than five-fold increase for 2–3 years after a severe head injury, but the excess risk continued for 10 years after mild (1.5 times) and severe brain injury (4.3 times), which is longer than that seen in Annegers et al. study. The relative risk increased with age for both mild and severe injuries and was especially high among people older than 15 years of age with mild (3.5 times) and severe (12.2 times) injury. The risk was slightly higher in women (2.5 times) than in men (2.0 times). The incidence of epilepsy was also greater in head injured people with a family history of epilepsy than in those without a family history, with about a six-fold increase in the relative risk of epilepsy after a mild head injury and a ten-fold increase after a severe injury. At 10 years after a severe TBI, even in individuals who had not by that time had a first unprovoked seizure, the risk of subsequently developing seizures/epilepsy was still on average at least four times higher (range 2.65–7.30, depending on other risk factors) than in noninjured individuals. Patients with a mild TBI were approximately 1.5 times more likely to develop epilepsy than patients without a TBI, but if they had not done so within 5 years, this risk no longer persisted.

This is a retrospective case study like that performed by Annegers and colleagues. This form of study produces inaccuracies with regards to the diagnosis of epilepsy and classification of head injury severity as it relies on unvalidated registry data for the diagnoses of both epilepsy and TBI. In addition, this study only included patients less than 26 years of age. However, the scale of the study (78,000 individuals with head injuries identified) makes this a valuable epidemiological assessment. This study found that the risk of epilepsy was increased for at least 10 years after head injury, even in mild cases. This is a longer period than that found by Annegers et al. This may be due to different study design and head injury severity classification, but even so, it highlights that post-traumatic epileptogenesis is a long process, which raises the possibility that neuroprotective measures could interfere with this process and thus reduce the risk of epilepsy.

Ferguson et al. conducted a prospective study of a sample of patients with a diagnosis of TBI who were discharged from hospital between 1999 and 2002.[14] Patients were older than 15 years of age and were interviewed yearly at 1, 2 and 3 years after discharge. In the first year interview, there were 2,118 persons with a TBI participating; this dropped to 1,536 by the second year and 1,173 by the third year. A total of 115 individuals were determined to have developed PTE within the 3 years of their hospital discharge. Patients were stratified into mild, moderate or severe injuries based on the head Abbreviated Injury Scale (AIS)[25] with mild = 2, moderate = 3 and severe = 4 or 5 (note an AIS score of 6 = death or critical injury with unlikely recovery and a score of 1 = no loss of consciousness but possible head injury). There was no control group for comparison.

The cumulative incidence of PTE in the first 3 years after discharge, after adjusting for loss to follow-up, was 4.4 per 100 persons over 3 years for hospitalized mild TBI, 7.6 for moderate and 13.6 for severe. Those with severe TBI, post-traumatic seizures prior to discharge and a history of depression were most at risk for PTE. This higher risk group also included persons with three or more chronic medical conditions at discharge.

In this study, TBI was defined as any hospital discharge with a primary or secondary diagnosis of trauma to the head associated with decreased consciousness, amnesia, other neurologic or neuropsychological abnormalities, skull fracture or intracranial lesion. As all the patients included in the study had been hospitalized, it is likely that there is a selection bias towards more severe injuries. The classification system used, the AIS, is different to that used in the previous two studies. The AIS is poorly correlated with other severity scales, e.g. GCS,[27] and only weakly correlated with outcome.[27] This study also has several design flaws; there was a large attrition rate of 45% over the 3 year follow-up, no data on key clinical markers including scan abnormalities and duration of loss of consciousness, and the methodology for identifying epilepsy may underestimate the incidence as it relied on self-report, assumed an absence of epilepsy where no data was collected and the insensitivity of the questions used to identify epilepsy. However, it sampled a large, demographically heterogeneous group of individuals who suffered a TBI and identified an association between depression and other medical co-morbidities with the risk of developing PTE.

Zhao et al. conducted a retrospective follow-up study of patients of all ages discharged from a brain injury centre in China with a diagnosis of a TBI between 2004 and 2008. TBI severity was based on GCS rating. Patients were followed-up via a telephone survey 3–5 years after the TBI. PTE was diagnosed after two or more unprovoked seizures. A total of 2,826 TBI patients were assessed, with 141 having a diagnosis of PTE. The incidence of epilepsy was not compared to a normative group and nor were rates corrected for other factors (e.g. co-morbid medical conditions).

The risk of development of PTE was 3.6%, 6.9% and 17% in the mild, moderate and severe categories respectively. Seventy-six per cent of patients developed seizures within the first year after the injury. Older age, severity of TBI, abnormal neuroimaging, surgical intervention and presence of early seizures were all identified as independent risk factors for later development of PTE. This was a relatively small study with no normative control group. Individuals all required inpatient care and so the mild group is likely to be relatively severe as most cases of mild TBI do not require inpatient care. Unlike previous studies, they identified early seizures as an independent risk factor for the later development of PTE, with two thirds of patients suffering early post-traumatic seizures going on to develop PTE.

Yeh et al. conducted a large retrospective population-based case-control study from Taiwan's National Health Institute Research Database.[30] They identified 19,336 patients who had suffered a TBI between 2000 and 2003 and followed them up until the end of 2008 (therefore follow-up period was 5–8 years). They compared to 540,322 matched controls who had not suffered a TBI. All patients were aged 15 or older. Patients were stratified based on the International Classification of Diseases, ninth edition (ICD-9-CM) into mild TBI (ICD-9-CM 850), severe TBI (ICD-9-CM 851–854) and presence of skull fracture(s) (ICD-9-CM 800–804). The difficulties with these classification criteria are discussed in the previous section.

Individuals who suffered a TBI had a higher incidence of low income, were less likely to live in an urban setting and had a higher risk of other medical problems. After adjusting for age, income, gender, urbanization and co-existing diseases, individuals with a skull fracture, severe TBI and mild TBI were 10.6, 5.1 and 3.0 times more likely to develop epilepsy respectively. This study showed that men had a greater risk of development of PTE compared to women (adjusted hazard ration 1.7) and that increasing age at time of TBI also conferred a greater risk. The risk was highest in the first year after injury but persisted for 4 years after a skull fracture or severe brain injury.

This is the largest retrospective study to date with a large normative control group. However, the risk of epilepsy is likely to be over-estimated in the mild group as it only included patients requiring emergency treatment and in-patient care and included patients with loss of consciousness greater than 24 hours. Additionally, there is a limited follow up period when previous studies suggest the risk can continue for decades. However, it again demonstrates in a large population that TBI is a sizeable risk factor for the development of epilepsy. It again shows that the risk is greatest soon after injury (i.e. within the first year) and that more severe injury with cerebral haemorrhage is associated with greater risk. It also identifies male gender and increasing age as separate risk factors but showed that the risk did not persist beyond 4 years after injury.

Mahler et al. conducted a population-based case-control study with an alternate design. They first identified 1,885 individuals of all ages with a validated unprovoked seizure and then determined the prevalence of TBI in this cohort compared to 15,080 matched controls.[29] Patients with a first unprovoked seizure were identified from a validated Swedish epilepsy register between 2000 and 2008. The Swedish National Inpatient Registry was then used to identify a hospital discharge diagnosis of a TBI in each group between 1980 and 2008. The ICD was used to classify TBI into skull fracture, mild and severe TBI in the same way as Yeh et al. They identified 105 patients with a TBI in the seizure group and 31 in the control group. Mild TBI was associated with a doubled risk for unprovoked seizures, skull fracture with a fourfold risk and severe TBI with an eight-fold risk. Age and gender did not have a significant effect on risk. Intracerebral haemorrhage and cerebral contusions were independent risk factors for increased seizure risk. The risk of seizure development was highest within the first 6 months after injury but the risk remained elevated for longer than 10 years in both the severe (2.2 times) and mild (2.0 times) TBI groups.

This is another large study using national registry data. It benefits from using an epilepsy registry with validated data, unlike the previous registry-based studies. Again, the TBI data relies on hospital discharge information and they use ICD classification, which is likely to result in more severe TBI cases being included in the mild group. Furthermore, patients with mild TBI often do not attend hospital and so the prevalence of PTE in the mild group is likely to be inflated.

Summary of Evidence

A TBI is a major risk factor for the future development of epilepsy. Severity of brain injury is a key factor in the likelihood of developing epilepsy, with up to a 17-fold increased risk in those suffering a severe closed head injury[1] and around a 50% risk associated with a penetrating injury.[21] Intracerebral contusions and subdural haematomas are also major risk factors for developing epilepsy.[1] Time after injury is also a critical factor when determining risk of developing PTE. The greatest risk occurs within the first year of injury and decreases rapidly over time, although a small risk persists for more than 10 years after a severe TBI. There is nearly a hundred-fold increased incidence within a year of a severe TBI, falling to four-fold after 10 years.[1]

Epidemiological studies also suggest even mild head injuries may confer an increased risk for the development of epilepsy. However, when interpreting this, it should be borne in mind that many people suffering a mild injury do not seek medical attention, and therefore there is a bias towards more severe injuries in the mild groups in these epidemiological studies. In addition, many of the epidemiological studies used classification systems that underestimate the severity, again inflating the risk for this group.

When counselling patients regarding the risk of epilepsy after a TBI, it is also important to take into account the absolute risk of seizures. Absolute risk depends upon numerous individual factors, including the nature of the injury, genetic predisposition, age, lifestyle factors, such as drug and alcohol use, and medical co-morbidities. Overall, the average annual incidence of epilepsy is predicted at around 0.05–0.055 %[33] in the general population. Therefore, within the first year of an injury around 5% of patients suffering a severe TBI are at risk of developing PTE, ~0.3% of patients suffering a moderate TBI and ~0.15% after a mild TBI as per the Annegers et al. classification.[1] Therefore, although even a mild TBI may confer a greater risk of future development of epilepsy, the absolute risk in this group is still at worst small.

It is also likely that genetic and other individual characteristics (such as additional medical co-morbidities) influence the risk of developing PTE.[14, 15]

Conclusions

A TBI is a clear risk factor for the development of epilepsy. The risk is greatest within the first year of an injury and decreases rapidly over time but an increased risk compared to the general population continues for many years. Severity of TBI is the biggest risk factor, with penetrating injuries and the presence of cerebral contusions and subdural haematomas being important clinical indicators of future risk. Individual characteristics including a family history of epilepsy, medical co-morbidities and a history of depression also seem to confer a greater risk. There is therefore an interplay between individual and injury factors in determining the future risk of developing PTE. Understanding these risks is important to allow accurate counselling of patients, directing treatment and making guidelines such as determining the risks of driving.

References

1. Annegers JF, Hauser WA, Coan SP, Rocca WA. A population-based study of seizures after traumatic brain injuries. *N Engl J Med* 1998; **338**: 20–4.

2. Asikainen I, Kaste M, Sarna S. Early and late posttraumatic seizures in traumatic brain injury rehabilitation patients: Brain injury factors causing late seizures and influence of seizures on long-term outcome. *Epilepsia* 1999; **40**: 584–9.

3. Englander J, Bushnik T, Wright JM, Jamison L, Duong TT. Mortality in late post-traumatic seizures. *J Neurotrauma* 2009; **26**: 1471–7.

4. Haltiner AM, Temkin NR, Dikmen SS. Risk of seizure recurrence after the first late posttraumatic seizure. *Arch Phys Med Rehabil* 1997; **78**: 835–40.

5. Maas AIR, Menon DK, Adelson PD, Andelic N, Bell MJ, Belli A, et al. Traumatic brain injury: integrated approaches to improve prevention, clinical care, and research. *Lancet Neurol* 2017; **16**: 987–1048.

6. Hauser WA, Annegers JF, Kurland LT. Incidence of epilepsy and unprovoked seizures in Rochester, Minnesota: 1935–1984. *Epilepsia* 1993; **34**: 453–68.

7. WHO. Epilepsy: a public health imperative: summary. World Health Organization, 2019.

8. Kotsopoulos IAW, van Merode T, Kessels FGH, de Krom MCTF, Knottnerus JA. Systematic review and meta-analysis of incidence studies of epilepsy and unprovoked seizures. *Epilepsia* 2002; **43**: 1402–9.

9. Hesdorffer DC, Logroscino G, Benn EKT, Katri N, Cascino G, Hauser WA. Estimating risk for developing epilepsy. *Neurology* 2011; **76**: 23–7.

10. Beghi E, Carpio A, Forsgren L, Hesdorffer DC, Malmgren K, Sander JW, et al. Recommendation for a definition of acute symptomatic seizure. *Epilepsia* 2010; **51**: 671–5.

11. Fisher RS, Acevedo C, Arzimanoglou A, Bogacz A, Cross JH, Elger CE, et al. ILAE Official Report: A practical clinical definition of epilepsy. *Epilepsia* 2014; **55**: 475–82.

12. Hauser WA, Rich SS, Lee JR, Annegers JF, Anderson VE. Risk of recurrent seizures after two unprovoked seizures. *N Engl J Med* 1998; **338**: 429–34.

13. van Diessen E, Lamberink HJ, Otte WM, Doornebal N, Brouwer OF, Jansen FE, et al. A prediction model to determine childhood epilepsy after 1 or more paroxysmal events. *Pediatrics* 2018; **142**: e20180931.

14. Ferguson PL, Smith GM, Wannamaker BB, Thurman DJ, Pickelsimer EE, Selassie AW. A population-based study of risk of epilepsy after hospitalization for traumatic brain injury. *Epilepsia* 2010; **51**: 891–8.

15. Christensen J, Pedersen MG, Pedersen CB, Sidenius P, Olsen J, Vestergaard M. Long-term risk of epilepsy after traumatic brain injury in children and young adults: a population-based cohort study. *Lancet* 2009; **373**: 1105–10.

16. Fisher RS, Boas WvE, Blume W, Elger C, Genton P, Lee P, et al. Epileptic seizures and epilepsy: Definitions Proposed by the International League Against Epilepsy (ILAE) and the International Bureau for Epilepsy (IBE). *Epilepsia* 2005; **46**: 470–2.

17. Berg AT. Risk of recurrence after a first unprovoked seizure. *Epilepsia* 2008; **49 Suppl 1**: 13–8.

18. Hesdorffer DC, Benn EK, Cascino GD, Hauser WA. Is a first acute symptomatic seizure epilepsy? Mortality and risk for recurrent seizure. *Epilepsia* 2009.

19. Fisher RS, Cross JH, French JA, Higurashi N, Hirsch E, Jansen FE, et al. Operational classification of seizure types by the International League Against Epilepsy: Position Paper of the ILAE Commission for Classification and Terminology. *Epilepsia* 2017; **58**: 522–30.

20. Scheffer IE, Berkovic S, Capovilla G, Connolly MB, French J, Guilhoto L, et al. ILAE classification of the epilepsies: Position paper of the ILAE Commission for Classification and Terminology. *Epilepsia* 2017; **58**: 512–21.

21. Salazar AM, Jabbari B, Vance SC, Grafman J, Amin D, Dillon JD. Epilepsy after penetrating head injury. I. Clinical correlates: a report of the Vietnam Head Injury Study. *Neurology* 1985; **35**: 1406–14.

22. Williams DH, Levin HS, Eisenberg HM. Mild head injury classification. *Neurosurgery* 1990; **27**: 422–8.

23. Malec JF, Brown AW, Leibson CL, Flaada JT, Mandrekar JN, Diehl NN, et al. The mayo classification system for traumatic brain injury severity. *J Neurotrauma* 2007; **24**: 1417–24.

24. Rimel RW, Giordani B, Barth JT, Jane JA. Moderate head injury: completing the clinical spectrum of brain trauma. *Neurosurgery* 1982; **11**: 344–51.

25. Association for the Advancement of Automotive Medicine, Committee on Injury Scaling. The Abbreviated Injury Scale, 1990 revision (AIS-90). Association for the Advancement of Automotive Medicine, Des Plaines, IL.

26. Foreman BP, Caesar RR, Parks J, Madden C, Gentilello LM, Shafi S, et al. Usefulness of the abbreviated injury score and the injury severity score in comparison to the Glasgow Coma Scale in predicting outcome after traumatic brain injury. *J Trauma* 2007; **62**: 946–50.

27. Demetriades D, Kuncir E, Murray J, Velmahos GC, Rhee P, Chan L. Mortality prediction of head Abbreviated Injury Score and Glasgow Coma Scale: analysis of 7,764 head injuries. *Journal of the American College of Surgeons* 2004; **199**: 216–22.

28. Walder AD, Yeoman PM, Turnbull A. The abbreviated injury scale as a predictor of outcome of severe head injury. *Intensive Care Med* 1995; **21**: 606–9.

29. Mahler B, Carlsson S, Andersson T, Adelow C, Ahlbom A, Tomson T. Unprovoked seizures after traumatic brain injury: A population-based case-control study. *Epilepsia* 2015; **56**: 1438–44.

30. Yeh CC, Chen TL, Hu CJ, Chiu WT, Liao CC. Risk of epilepsy after traumatic brain injury: a retrospective population-based cohort study. *J Neurol Neurosurg Psychiatry* 2013; **84**: 441–5.

31. Sharp DJ, Jenkins PO. Concussion is confusing us all. *Pract Neurol* 2015; **15**: 172–86.

32. Frey LC. Epidemiology of posttraumatic epilepsy: A critical review. *Epilepsia* 2003; **44**: 11–7.

33. Forsgren L, Beghi E, Oun A, Sillanpaa M. The epidemiology of epilepsy in Europe – a systematic review. *Eur J Neurol* 2005; **12**: 245–53.

34. Zhao Y, Wu H, Wang X, Li J, Zhang S. Clinical epidemiology of posttraumatic epilepsy in a group of Chinese patients. *Seizure* 2012; **21**:322–6.

Chapter 3

Traumatic Brain Injury: The Acute Management and Prevention Programmes

Colette Griffin

Introduction

The last decade in the UK has seen improvements in the way that traumatic brain injury (TBI) is managed, with the implementation of Major Trauma Networks. Enhanced pre-hospital approaches, excellent leadership, standardised care and governance are some of the reasons a patient is 30% more likely to survive major trauma today in the UK.[1]

The recent Lancet Neurology Commission on TBI highlighted the scope and considerable public health challenge of TBI. It estimated that 50% of the world's population will experience one or more traumatic brain injury in their lifetime.[2] The Commission particularly highlighted the urgent need for the development, validation and implementation of prognostic models in TBI, particularly less severe TBI; 80–90% of all TBI cases fall into less severe classifications.[3]

The Collaborative European NeuroTrauma Effectiveness Research in Traumatic Brain Injury (CENTER-TBI) core study is a European Commission funded observational study that began in 2013. It aims to characterise TBI, identify best practices, develop precision medicine and improve outcomes via comparative-effectiveness studies. The CENTER-TBI study is closely linked with the US Transforming Research and Clinical Knowledge in Traumatic Brain Injury (TRACK-TBI) study and forms part of a franchise of studies making up the International Initiative for Traumatic Brain Injury Research (InTBIR). Therefore the findings of CENTRE-TBI will be greatly amplified by analyses across the InTBIR studies.

Early neurorehabilitation in TBI has been shown to shorten overall hospital stay, reduce the likelihood of being discharged into a care setting and improve functional outcomes at one year.[4] The development of TBI neurorehabilitation facilities collocated within Major Trauma Centres should therefore be a priority in ongoing TBI service redesign.

Facilitating individualised management of TBI to optimise diagnosis, track disease progression and improve outcome prediction is the pathway of the future for TBI. There is therefore an unmet medical need for rapid blood-based biomarker tests, as an adjunct to imaging studies.

Substantial scientific advances in the past decade have resulted in identification of blood-based protein biomarkers that are relevant to different phases of TBI.[5, 6] Ongoing research efforts are yielding new classes of biomarkers, including metabolic and lipid markers, microRNAs and exosomes.[7–9] These hold potential for diagnosis, prognosis and therapeutic stratification, but are not yet in advanced clinical development.

Epidemiology

Approximately 50 million people worldwide each year sustain a TBI, and the cost is estimated as being 0.5% of global economic output.[10] The incidence, including the whole range of TBI severity from minor to very severe injuries, varies in different countries, from 60 cases per 100,000 inhabitants up to numbers 12 times higher.[11] This reflects local variations, varying diagnostic criteria and methodologies. There are an estimated one million A&E attendances in the UK each year due to TBI.[12] TBI is the single largest cause of death and disability in the under 40-year-old age group.

The number of TBI admissions in the UK in 2015 had increased by 6% compared to 2005–2006, and males were 1.6 times more likely to sustain a TBI than females.[13] Calls to the Headway charity nurse-led helpline also increased by 60% between 2010 and 2014. Of particular note, the data showed a 61% increase in the incidence of TBI in the female population, when compared to 2000–2001. This may be due to multiple factors such as increased life expectancy, increased alcohol consumption and potentially increased risk-taking behaviour in the female population.

It is estimated that TBI costs £15 billion per year in the UK through direct and indirect costs.[10] TBI is known to reduce life expectancy and is also a risk factor for premature death and suicide.[14] It doubles the risk of developing a mental health disorder,[15] and it is estimated that 50% of adults and 33% of young offenders in prison have a history of a TBI.[16] In addition to the impact of TBI on the individual and their family, the societal costs can be substantial. In the UK, health and social care costs for people with TBI have been estimated at £71.1 million for the 18–25-year-old age group alone.[17]

Figures regarding the prevalence of people living with the consequences of TBI are less well documented. It has been estimated, however, that millions of people (approximately five million in the USA and seven million in Europe) were living with TBI-related disability in 2014.[18]

Epidemiological studies also show increased mortality rates even after a mild traumatic brain injury. One large cohort study showed that 15 years after the injury, the mortality rate in young patients with a mild TBI was higher than the rate in matched controls.[19] Patients with mild TBI had higher mortality rates than those with other types of injury, so the findings were not due to nonspecific lifestyle factors associated with those exposing themselves to potential injury.

Classification

Severity classification in TBI has been of interest due to its relationship to outcome and post-acute medical care.[20] TBI severity can be classified both for clinical and research purposes using single indicators, such as duration of post traumatic amnesia (PTA),[21] duration of loss of consciousness,[22] and Glasgow Coma Scale (GCS),[23] or a combination of the above (see Table 3.1).

Although these measures are well established, they may be influenced by other factors such as sedation, intoxication and psychological shock. Whilst neuroimaging provides an objective anatomical indicator of severity,[24] it is often not obtained in the less severe cases.

With the advent of neuroimaging, it has become increasingly possible to classify TBI in a clinical setting on a pathoanatomic basis, where the features and location of traumatic abnormalities can be defined both from clinical features and radiological appearances.

Table 3.1 The Mayo classification system

Mayo TBI Severity Classification System

A. Classify as Moderate-Severe (Definite) TBI if one or more of the following criteria apply:

1. Death due to this TBI

2. Loss of consciousness of 30 minutes or more

3. Post-traumatic anterograde amnesia of 24 hours or more

4. Worst Glasgow Coma Scale full score in first 24 hours <13 (unless invalidated upon review)

5. One or more of the following present:

• Intracerebral haematoma

• Subdural haematoma

• Cerebral contusion

• Haemorrhagic contusion

• Penetrating TBI (dura penetrated)

• Subarachnoid haemorrhage

• Brain stem injury

B. If none of Criteria A apply, classify as Mild (probable) TBI if 1 or more of the following apply:

1. Loss of consciousness of momentary to less than 30 minutes

2. Post-traumatic anterograde amnesia of momentary to less than 24 hours

3. Depressed, basilar, or linear skull fracture (dura intact)

C. If none of Criteria A or B apply, classify as Symptomatic (Possible) TBI if 1 or more of the following are present:

• Blurred vision

• Confusion (mental state changes)

• Dazed

• Dizziness

• Focal neurologic symptoms

• Headache

• Nausea

Pathoanatomic features may be a more important determinant of long-term neuropsychological outcome than classifications based on severity, as defined by clinical factors alone.

Different imaging modalities are available to classify TBI, with CT being most commonly used in the acute traumatic presentation. MRI is used further down the line of recovery to guide prognosis and diagnosis of pathologies, such as diffuse axonal injury. This is often difficult to diagnose on initial CT imaging.[25] Other imaging modalities such as diffusion tensor imaging,[26] functional MRI[27] and PET imaging[28] are currently promising research tools but are not widely used in day-to-day clinical practice.

Acute Management

The ideal management of patients with an acute TBI allows accurate and timely diagnosis of the complex problems which occur both immediately and less acutely post-TBI. It should also provide rapid and accurate treatment, and it should be focused on pathological and impairment based diagnostics and therapeutics.

Stroke services are now organised into Hyper Acute Stroke Units and Stroke Units, with all stroke patients being cared for by a Stroke Consultant on a dedicated and specialist stroke ward. This is currently not the case for TBI patients in many countries. Cohorting patients who have suffered a stroke has been shown to increase cohesion of the care pathway, improve patient flow, reduce preventable disability and reduce length of stay.[29]

Major Trauma Networks were developed in order to get the right patient to the right place at the right time. Progress has been made in identifying and treating, in a timely fashion, secondary insults to the brain including hypoxia, hypotension, seizures and intracranial haematomas.

Pre-hospital TBI care has greatly improved over the past few decades.[30] This care has emphasised rapid, safe extrication of the trauma victim, stabilisation of the spine, aggressive resuscitation to prevent hypotension, immediate airway management and rapid, safe transport to an appropriate trauma centre. The most important key feature of current paediatric and adult head injury protocols is the aim to decrease all potential secondary brain insults.

The early detection of an intracranial haematoma would allow focusing of the trauma pathway on the needs of the individual patient. Therefore, access to better monitoring at the roadside is desirable. If patients survive the first few minutes, there is a therapeutic window of opportunity to intervene and prevent further death of brain tissue.

Currently, TBI is managed uniformly. The pre-hospital data field does not specify the type of brain injury, if any. Hence all such patients receive the same treatment (usually intubation and transfer to a neurosurgical unit). On-scene diagnosis of injury would permit more directed therapies to be initiated. It is vital to dispatch resources appropriate for the presumed severity of injury. Currently pre-hospital dispatch criteria are often based on 'mechanism of injury' (e.g. fall > 2 floors, ejected from car) and interrogation of emergency line callers.

Different types of traumatic intracranial bleeding (haematomas) exist, all of which can compress the brain and can be life-threatening. Timely surgery can be life-saving, but this depends on rapid patient transfer to a centre with neurosurgical facilities. Initial neurosurgical treatment of TBI can be either causally directed (e.g. to remove space-occupying intracranial haematomas)[31] or symptomatic (e.g. to decrease pressure on the brain to prevent or minimise damage to important structures and prevent life-threatening herniation events). Symptomatic approaches include insertion of an external ventricular drain for drainage of cerebrospinal fluid[32, 33] and decompressive craniectomy, which can be performed in the same setting as the evacuation of a haematoma, or later to treat diffuse brain swelling that is refractory to conservative medical management.

Substantial variation exists in neurosurgical practice, owing to an inadequate evidence base for international guidelines on surgical indications.[34–36] Additionally, at the level of individual patients, there is debate among clinicians regarding which patients might benefit from some procedures, such as surgical treatment for traumatic intracranial lesions and for raised intracranial pressure (ICP), and uncertainty regarding the optimum timing of surgery.

Surgery might be life-saving and preserve neurological function in some patients,[37] but others might survive with an unfavourable functional outcome, ranging from severe neurological and cognitive deficits to a vegetative state.[38–40] Conversely, surgery might not always be necessary. A substantial proportion of patients who are managed conservatively have favourable outcomes.[41–45]

Therefore, when deciding whether to operate, medical therapies that might be effective in achieving the same physiological goals as surgery should also be considered. Surgical indications that are too liberal could lead to increased survival with complications of unnecessary surgery in patients with less severe injury, or severe disabilities in those with devastating TBI.

Conversely, inappropriate conservative management might result in unnecessary death and disability. The decision to operate is based not only on medical but also on ethical considerations. Patients' and relatives' views of a meaningful quality of life might be different from the medical perception of a favourable outcome. These differences could depend on several factors, including cultural and religious considerations. If discussion of the expected outcome with relatives is possible, past views expressed by patients on an acceptable quality of life should be taken into consideration.[46]

Accumulating evidence provides useful support for such decision making. An illustrative example is the use of decompressive craniectomy for intracranial hypertension. Although the procedure can be life-saving by lowering ICP, it is often associated with surgical complications, and structural distortions associated with removal of a portion of the skull might cause additional brain injury in some patients.[47] Initially used over a century ago, the intervention has come back into use over the past two decades, but given the need to balance risks and benefits, a clear definition of its role has been difficult.[48–50]

Two important randomised control trials (RCTs) have provided useful guidance in this context. The DECRA (Decompressive Craniectomy) trial showed that very early use of decompressive craniectomy for modest rises in ICP in patients with diffuse injuries was associated with worse outcomes.[51] More recently, the RESCUEicp (Randomised Evaluation of Surgery with Craniectomy for Uncontrollable Elevation of Intracranial Pressure) trial showed that, when used for refractory severe intracranial hypertension, decompressive craniectomy could save lives, but resulted in a 9% increase in survival with severe dependence at 6 months.[52] However, by 12 months, there were 13% more survivors who were at least independent at home. As the intervention is not uniformly beneficial, individual wishes of patients and their families should be taken into consideration.

Other studies have addressed similar surgical dilemmas. A recent study suggested that in patients with a traumatic acute subdural haemorrhage, early evacuation was associated with better outcome than a more conservative approach.[53] Similar trends were noted in the STITCH (Surgical Trial In Traumatic intraCerebral Haemorrhage) study[54] which reported better outcomes with early surgical management in patients with traumatic intracerebral haemorrhage. However, the results of the STITCH trial were not statistically significant owing to an inadequate sample size caused by premature discontinuation of the trial by the funding agency.[55] The RESCUE-ASDH (Randomised Evaluation of Surgery with Craniectomy for patients Undergoing Evacuation of Acute SubDural Haematoma) trial is currently ongoing. Clinical decision making could be greatly improved by the identification of patient subgroups most likely to benefit from the intervention and, importantly, patients who are not likely to benefit.

The consequences of TBI either arise as a primary consequence of the trauma (through direct contact and/or through acceleration–deceleration forces) or secondary to subsequent nontraumatic consequences. The injuries may be focal, diffuse, or both. Focal injuries include skull fractures, haemorrhage and contusions. Diffuse injuries include diffuse axonal injury (DAI) and/or vascular injury.[56]

Intraparenchymal haemorrhage or intracerebral haemorrhage refers to significant bleeding within the brain parenchyma. Pathologically, contusions and intraparenchymal haematomas exist along the same continuum. In a contusion, blood is intermixed with brain tissue.[57] Radiologically, a contusion becomes an intraparenchymal haematoma once two thirds or more of the lesion is blood.[58]

Up to one third of all contusions enlarge in the subacute phase and so the extent of damage may be underestimated or missed on scans conducted immediately after the initial injury. A metabolic reaction is triggered in adjacent tissue, which peaks approximately 5 days after the injury. Mechanically, the inferior surfaces of both the frontal and temporal lobes are particularly vulnerable to contusional injury following TBI, due to the irregular bony surface floor of the frontal and middle cranial fossa. Injuries to the parenchyma in these regions can lead to persistent focal neuropsychological deficits.

The prognosis associated with extradural and subdural haemorrhages is improved if the injury is not associated with significant pressure effects, if there is no oedematous or inflammatory response in the underlying parenchyma and if the haemorrhage does not require surgical management.

However, the risk of morbidity and mortality increases significantly if the bleed requires surgical intervention, particularly if this is delayed.[59] Mass effects are better tolerated in some brain regions than others. Figure 3.1 shows a large acute extradural haemorrhage requiring urgent neurosurgical intervention.

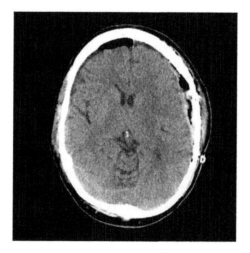

Figure 3.1 An acute left sided extradural haematoma with midline shift and uncal herniation requiring urgent neurosurgical intervention.

Intraventricular haemorrhage can occur as a result of trauma, most commonly developing from a primary traumatic subarachnoid bleed. When associated with raised intracranial pressure, survivors of such injuries are at high risk of being left with significant and widespread cognitive difficulties.

Secondary injuries refer to the cerebral damage caused by events following the primary injury. These may occur as a direct consequence of the pathophysiological cascade triggered by the primary injury, or they may be the neurological consequences of other physical injuries sustained in the trauma. Secondary injuries can result from hypoxia, raised ICP, hypercarbia, hyponatraemia and seizures. The presence of any of these processes significantly increases the likelihood of developing long-term neurological sequelae following a TBI. The impact is cumulative, with the more injuries sustained by the brain, the less likely the patient is to make a full neurological recovery.

Cognitive deficits post-TBI commonly include reduced speed of cognitive processing, difficulties in memory and attention,[60, 61] language and executive functions.[62] Behavioural alterations such as impulsivity and aggression,[63] in addition to neuropsychiatric consequences, including depression and apathy, are commonly encountered.[64] There is also an increased rate of relationship breakdown amongst families coping with the effects of TBI.[65] Other areas that are frequently affected are social reintegration and life satisfaction,[66] educational attainment[67] and vocational outcome.[68]

The resolution of confusion or PTA immediately post-TBI is often commonly followed by a constellation of symptoms including dizziness, fatigue, headaches, reduced concentration, memory impairment, sleep disturbance, irritability, photophobia, phonophobia, depression and blurred vision.

Most patients sustaining a mild TBI should be expected to recover within the first three months.[69] There are well documented factors that may cause this period of recovery to lengthen.[70] Up to one third of such patients report symptoms lasting up to six months.[71] The presence of a more severe initial injury, older age, female sex, previous head injuries and pre-existing psychological problems all make symptoms more likely to be persistent.[72]

Following the initial traumatic event, patients go through a long and complex process of functional recovery. There is a general trend for patients to experience an initial stage of rapid improvement, gradually plateauing over a period of two years.[73, 74]

Neurorehabilitation consists of a series of interventions tailored to the individual's unique bio-psycho-social needs, in order to optimise recovery and maximise functional outcomes. The ultimate aim of neurorehabilitation is to enhance community reintegration. In the UK, TBI hyper-acute neurorehabilitation may start following admission to intensive care, continuing into the community and vocational settings.

The point at which to commence intensive neurorehabilitation is a matter of ongoing debate. Introducing neurorehabilitation when patients remain in PTA with reduced physical and cognitive tolerance of therapy may be considered a misallocation of resources, but intervening too late may also have a negative impact on recovery.

Early (<35 days post injury) TBI rehabilitation admission leads to a significant reduction in length of intervention and total hospital stay, thus decreasing the associated cost of care.[75]

A prospective randomised study of a specialist multidisciplinary domiciliary outreach team showed that treatment increased independence and lessened care needs significantly when compared to standard care.[76] Residential neurorehabilitation for patients with neurobehavioural disorders after TBI improves functional outcomes and is estimated to result in lifetime savings of up to £1.13 million.[77]

PTA length can be used as an indicator of injury severity and has been shown to have prognostic value for long-term functional outcomes.[78, 79] There have been attempts to influence the length of PTA in order to improve TBI outcomes has been attempted.[80, 81] However, there is limited evidence for the effectiveness of early intervention in patients with PTA.[82]

A recent survey identified that fewer than 20% of neurotrauma centres have evidence-based guidance on the characteristics of intensive rehabilitation.[83] It is likely that progress in this domain has been hindered by the difficulties associated with conducting rigorous trials on complex interventions, particularly where doing so would involve delaying access to necessary interventions. Whilst recent progress has been made in quantifying the clinical and cost-effectiveness of parameters such as the number of disciplines involved and intervention intensity, evidence on optimal timing of neurorehabilitation is still scarce.[84, 85]

Long-term sequelae of TBI can include post traumatic headaches, seizures and neuro-degeneration. There is an increased incidence of Parkinson's disease[86] Alzheimer's disease,[87] and chronic traumatic encephalopathy.[88]

Prevention

Most TBIs are preventable, and the demographics are changing. Whilst TBI from high velocity injuries in young males still occur, the burgeoning elderly population with TBIs from falls from standing is increasing considerably.[89] The global ageing population is increasing in size dramatically. Altered physiology, anatomy, comorbidity and medications can influence the response to trauma and its medical management. There are also more TBIs occurring in several developing countries due to increased motorisation.

According to the World Health Organization (WHO), road traffic accidents are the number one cause of death among those aged 15–29 years, killing almost 1·3 million people of all ages each year. Approximately half of those killed are pedestrians, cyclists and motorcyclists.[90] Ninety percent of all TBI-related deaths occur in low and middle income countries.[91] Road traffic accident and trauma-related TBIs are increasing in these countries.

Only 28 countries, representing 449 million people (7% of the world's population), have adequate laws that address all of the top five risk factors for injury and premature death: seat belt use, child restraint use, speeding laws, drink driving laws and the use of a protective helmet. Road traffic injuries are currently estimated to be the ninth leading cause of death globally, and they are predicted to become the fifth leading cause of death by 2030.[90]

Among the people most at risk of sustaining a TBI are those using powered two-wheel vehicles. Mandatory helmet use has decreased the number and severity of head injuries among both motorcycle[92] and bicycle users.[93–95] In Taiwan, introduction of the motorcycle helmet law in 1997 reduced motorcycle-related head injuries by 33%, and injuries that did occur were less severe and were associated with shorter hospital stays.[96] Despite strong evidence that helmets reduce the severity of injuries from motorcycle crashes and increase the likelihood of survival, helmet laws are not universally implemented.[97]

The impact is greatest in low and middle income countries, where helmet wearing rates are only slightly above zero. Child passengers rarely wear helmets and those who do often wear adult helmets, offering inadequate protection. Where mandatory helmet laws are enacted, strong enforcement has yielded a 40% reduction in the risk of death.[90]

In high income countries, recent attention has focused on the risks incurred by distracted drivers.[98] The likelihood of a safety critical event occurring while driving has been reported to be six times higher for drivers dialling a mobile phone and 23 times higher for those texting. Although campaigns aimed at influencing drivers' behaviour remain relevant, technological solutions should also be considered. There have been suggestions to develop smart solutions to recognise and block nonhands-free mobile phone use whilst driving.

Annually, more than 600,000 individuals worldwide die from falls, the majority from TBI. The US Centre for Disease Control and Prevention reported that, in 2013, nearly 80% of all TBI-related Accident and Emergency department visits, hospital admissions, and deaths in adults aged 65 years and older were caused by falls.[99, 100]

The incidence of falls in low and middle income countries is likely to be underreported, and therefore, the global incidence of fall-related TBI is likely to be much higher than suggested by current estimates.

Crucial to improving TBI outcomes are pre-hospital emergency care at the scene of the injury, acute hospital inpatient care and post-acute care. The latter of these is rarely available in low resource settings. While 85% of high income countries have an emergency specialty for doctors, a recent WHO systematic review of emergency care in 59 low and middle income countries reported that only 28% of facilities had Consultant-level Physicians available full-time; 18% were staffed by specialty trained Accident and Emergency Physicians, and in only 4% were these available at all times.[101]

Therefore General Practitioners, Medical Practitioners and nurses, often without proper training, are often left to manage acute trauma. Furthermore, many patients with TBI require emergency neurosurgical intervention that is frequently non existent. In many countries in Africa, for example, the ratio of neurosurgeons to members of the population in 2005 was roughly 1 to 9 million.[102]

The UN has developed Sustainable Development Goals (SDGs), and SDG 3.6 aims to halve global deaths and injuries from road traffic accidents and ensure universal health coverage, by 2030.

Prevention initiatives can be applied at a population level with legislation, improvements in infrastructure, vehicle safety design, trauma care and workplace safety measures. Alternatively, prevention measures can focus on high risk subgroups. Examples include the targeting of drivers and cyclists to prevent alcohol impaired driving, speeding and distracted driving: promotion of seat belt, child restraint and helmet use; a focus on elderly people living alone and at risk of falls (see Figure 3.2) and strategies aimed at children at risk of abuse.

Prevention strategies need to take account of changing epidemiological patterns, which show increases in fall-related TBI in older individuals.[103–105] Frail elderly people are more likely to fall, more likely to suffer a TBI when a fall occurs and more likely to suffer long-term adverse effects even from a seemingly mild TBI.[106]

It might also be possible to specifically target individuals to address their patterns of risk-taking behaviour.[107] Irrespective of the target population, information campaigns should employ a range of measures to raise awareness of key issues in prevention and care for TBI. The potential of broad education and awareness campaigns, also using social media, is exemplified by the success of the ThinkFirst National Injury Prevention Foundation, established in the USA in 1990.[108]

Several studies have identified increased age as a factor prognostic of mortality following TBI.[109–111] Adults aged 65 years and over made more than 3.5 million visits to Accident and Emergency departments in England during the financial year 2012–2013.[100] Attendances by

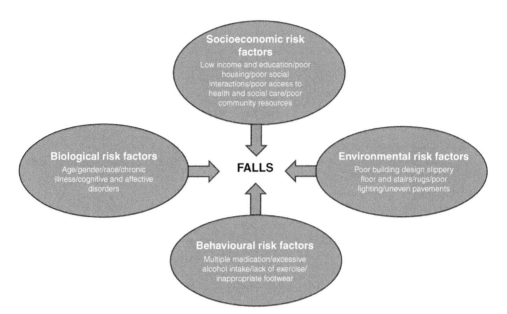

Figure 3.2 Falls in the elderly population are usually multifactorial.

this age group formed 19% of the 18.3 million Accident and Emergency department attendances in England that year.

Professional sports organisations are increasingly obliged to remove any player with a suspected TBI from play immediately, thus setting an example for amateur athletes and, in particular, young players. Such decisions should not be taken by interested parties (e.g. coaches), but rather by a neutral party such as an independent healthcare professional. The English Rugby Football Union has developed the widely publicised 'Headcase' project, and the SCAT 3 is used as a pitch side concussion detection programme.[112]

Various international efforts have been initiated to develop, refine and implement rational guidance for players, parents and coaches about the time that needs to be spent away from training and contact sport following a mild TBI.[113] However, further refinement in diagnosis is needed, as is guidance on action required when a mild TBI is reliably diagnosed.[114, 115]

In children and adolescents, there are additional concerns about the cumulative effects of multiple mild TBIs on brain development and learning, and the consequent cognitive and behavioural sequelae.[116] Children and young adults are also at increased risk of second impact syndrome.[117, 118]

Sport-related TBIs have received significant media coverage in recent years, in part due to an increased body of scientific literature and growing concern surrounding their long-term effects. The major focus is on mild TBI, as these account for 80% of TBI related visits to Accident and Emergency departments.

With the development and application of advanced mild TBI assessment tools, including neuropsychological testing, neuroimaging and balance and gait assessments, there is a rising tide of data that is driving changes in clinical practices and the management of patients with mild TBI.

References

1. Hawley C, Sakr M, Scapinello S, et al. Traumatic brain injuries in older adults—6 years of data for one UK trauma centre: retrospective analysis of prospectively collected data. *Emerg Med J* 2017;**34**:509–16.

2. Maas AIR, Menon DK, Adelson PD, et al. Traumatic brain injury: integrated approaches to improve prevention, clinical care and research. *Lancet Neurol* 2017;**16**:987–1048.

3. Saatman KE, Duhaime AC, Bullock R, et al. Classification of traumatic brain injury for targeted therapies. *J Neurotrauma* 2008;**25**:719–38.

4. Andelic N, Bautz-Holter E, Ronning P, et al. Does an early onset and continuous chain of rehabilitation improve the long term functional outcome of patients with severe traumatic brain injury? *J Neurotrauma* 2012;**29(1)**:66–74.

5. Rubenstein R, Chang B, Davies, et al. A novel, ultrasensitive assay for tau: potential for assessing traumatic brain injury in tissues and biofluids. *J Neurotrauma* 2015;**32**:342–52.

6. Shahim P, Tegner Y, Wilson DHD, et al. Blood biomarkers for brain injury in concussed professional ice hockey players. *JAMA Neurol* 2014;**71**:684–92.

7. Mitra B, Rau TF, Surendran N, et al. Plasma micro-RNA biomarkers for diagnosis and prognosis after traumatic brain injury: a pilot study. *J Clin Neurosci* 2017;**38**:37–42.

8. Posti JP, Dickens AM, Orešič M, et al. Metabolomics profiling as a diagnostic tool in severe traumatic brain injury. *Front Neurol* 2017;**8**:398.

9. Martínez-Morillo E, Childs C, García BP, et al. Neurofilament medium polypeptide (NFM) protein concentration is increased in CSF and serum samples from patients with brain injury. *Clin Chem Lab Med* 2015;**53**:1575–84.

10. Engberg AW, Teasdale TW. Psychosocial outcome following traumatic brain injury in adults: a long-term population based follow up. *Brain Injury* 2013;**27**:1500–7.

11. Feigin VL, Theadom A, Barker-Collo S, et al. Incidence of traumatic brain injury in New Zealand: a population based study. *Lancet Neurol* 2013;**12(1)**:53–64.

12. Kay A, Teasdale G. Head injury in the United Kingdom. *World J Surg* 2001;**25**:1210–20.

13. Tennant A 2015. www.headway.org.uk/media/2883/acquired-brain-injury-the-numbers-behind-the-hidden-disability.pdf

14. McMillan TM, Teasdale GM, Weir CJ, et al. Death after head injury: the 13 year outcome of a case control study. *J Neurol Neurosurg Psychiatry* 2011;**82**:931–5.

15. Williams MW, Rapport LJ, Millis SR, et al. Psychosocial outcomes after traumatic brain injury: life satisfaction, community integration, and distress. *Rehabil Psychol* 2014;**59(3)**:298–305.

16. Parsonage M. Traumatic Brain Injury and Offending: an economic analysis. *Barrow and Cadbury Trust Centre for Mental Health* July 2016.

17. Beecham J, Perkins M, Snell T, et al. Treatment paths and costs for young adults with acquired brain injury in the United Kingdom. *Brain Inj* 2009;**23**(1):30–8.

18. Ponsford JL, Downing MG, Olver, J, et al. Longitudinal follow-up of patients with traumatic brain injury: outcome at two, five, and ten years post-injury. *J Neurotrauma* 2014;**31(1)**:64–77.

19. McMillan TM, Weir CJ, Wainman-Lefley J. Mortality and morbidity 15 years after hospital admission with mild traumatic brain injury: a prospective case-controlled population study. *J Neurol Neurosurg Psychiatry* 2014;**85**:1214–20.

20. Levin HS. Prediction of recovery from traumatic brain injury. *J Neurotrauma* 1995;**12**:913–22.

21. Brown AW, Malec JF, McClelland RL, et al. Clinical elements that predict outcome after traumatic brain injury: a prospective multicentre recursive partitioning (decision-tree) analysis. *J Neurotrauma* 2005;**22**:1040–51.

22. Whyte J, Cifu D, Dikmen S, et al. Prediction of functional outcomes after traumatic brain injury: a comparison of 2 measures of duration of unconsciousness. *Arch Phys Med Rehabil* 2001;**82**:1355–9.

23. Zafonte RD, Hammond FM, Mann NR, et al. Relationship between Glasgow Coma Scale and functional outcome. *Am J Phys Med Rehabil* 1996;**75**:364–9.

24. Marshall LF, Marshall SB, Klauber MR, et al. The diagnosis of head injury requires a classification based on computed axial tomography. *J Neurotrauma* 1992;**9(suppl 1)**:S287–92.

25. Scheid R, Preul C, Gruber O, et al. Diffuse axonal injury associated with chronic traumatic brain injury: evidence from T2* weighted gradient-echo imaging at 3T. *AJNR Am J Neuroradiol* 2003;**24**:1049–56.

26. Sidaros A, Engberg AW, Sidaros K, et al. Diffusion tensor imaging during recovery from severe traumatic brain injury and relation to clinical outcome: a longitudinal study. *Brain* 2008;**131**:559–72.

27. McAllister TW, Saykin AJ, Flashman LA, et al. Brain activation during working memory 1 month after mild traumatic brain injury: a functional MRI study. *Neurology* 1999;**53**:1300–8.

28. Zhang J, Mitsis EM, Chu K, et al. Statistical parametric mapping and cluster counting analysis of[18F] FDG-PET imaging in traumatic brain injury *J Neurotrauma* 2010;**27**:35–49.

29. Hanger C, Fletcher V, Fink J, et al. Improving care for stroke patients: adding an acute stroke unit helps. *NZ Med J* 2007;**120(1250)**:2450.

30. Mate K, Williams D. Enhancing prehospital emergency care. *Healthcare Executive.* 2014;**29(5)**:64–7.

31. Bullock M, Chesnut R, Ghajar J. Guidelines for the surgical management of traumatic brain injury. *Neurosurgery.* 2006;**58**:1–62.

32. Timofeev I, Dahyot-Fizelier C, Keong N, et al. Ventriculostomy for control of raised ICP in acute traumatic brain injury. *Acta Neurochir Suppl (Wien).* 2008;**102**:99–104.

33. Liu H, Wang W, Cheng F, et al. External ventricular drains versus intraparenchymal intracranial pressure monitors in traumatic brain injury: a prospective observational study. *World Neurosurg.* 2015;**83**:794–800.

34. Van Essen TA, de Ruiter GC, Kho KH, et al. Neurosurgical treatment variation of traumatic brain injury: evaluation of acute subdural hematoma management in Belgium and The Netherlands. *J Neurotrauma* 2017;**34**:881–9.

35. Compagnone C, Murray GD, Teasdale GM, et al. The management of patients with intradural post-traumatic mass lesions: a multicenter survey of current approaches to surgical management in 729 patients coordinated by the European Brain Injury Consortium. *Neurosurgery* 2005;**57**: 1183–92.

36. Ghajar J, Hariri RJ, Narayan RK, et al. Survey of critical care management of comatose, head-injured patients in the United States. *Crit Care Med* 1995;**23**: 560–7.

37. Seelig JM, Becker DP, Miller JD, et al. Traumatic acute subdural hematoma: major mortality reduction in comatose patients treated within four hours. *N Engl J Med* 1981;**304**:1511–18.

38. Tallon JM, Ackroyd-Stolarz S, Karim SA, et al. The epidemiology of surgically treated acute subdural and epidural hematomas in patients with head injuries: a population-based study. *Can J Surg* 2008;**51**:339–45.

39. Li LM, Kolias AG, Guilfoyle MR, et al. Outcome following evacuation of acute subdural haematomas: a comparison of craniotomy with decompressive craniectomy. *Acta Neurochir (Wien)* 2012;**154**:1555–61.

40. Nijboer JMM, van der Naalt J, Duis HJ. Patients beyond salvation? Various categories of trauma patients with a minimal Glasgow Coma Score. *Injury* 2010;**41**:52–7.

41. Dent DL, Croce MA, Menke PG, et al. Prognostic factors after acute subdural hematoma. *J Trauma* 1995;**39**: 36–42.

42. Mathew P, Oluoch-Olunya DL, Condon BR, et al. Acute subdural haematoma in the conscious patient: outcome with initial non-operative management. *Acta Neurochir (Wien)* 1993;**121**:100–8.

43. Servadei F, Nasi MT, Cremonini AM, et al. Importance of a reliable admission Glasgow Coma Scale score for determining the need for evacuation of post traumatic subdural hematomas: a prospective study of 65 patients. *J Trauma* 1998;**44**:868–73.

44. Wang R, Li M, Gao WW, et al. Outcomes of early decompressive craniectomy versus conventional medical management after severe traumatic brain injury: a systematic review and meta-analysis. *Medicine (Baltimore)* 2015; **94**:e1733.

45. Chang EF, Meeker M, Holland MC. Acute traumatic intraparenchymal haemorrhage: risk factors for progression in the early post-injury period. *Neurosurgery* 2006;**58**:647–56.

46. Cai X, Robinson J, Muehlschlegel S, et al. Patient preferences and surrogate decision making in neuroscience intensive care units. *Neurocrit Care* 2015;**23**:131–41.

47. Yang XF, Wen L, Shen F, et al. Surgical complications secondary to decompressive craniectomy in patients with a head injury: a series of 108 consecutive cases. *Acta Neurochir (Wien)* 2008;**150**:1241–7.

48. Servadei F, Compagnone C, Sahuquillo J. The role of surgery in traumatic brain injury. *Curr Opin Crit Care* 2007;**13**:163–8.

49. Honeybul S, Janzen C, Kruger K, et al. Decompressive craniectomy for severe traumatic brain injury: is life worth living? *J Neurosurg.* 2013;**119**:1566–75.

50. Guerra WK, Gaab MR, Dietz H, et al. Surgical decompression for traumatic brain swelling: indications and results. *J Neurosurg* 1999;**90**:187–96.

51. Cooper DJ, Rosenfeld JV, Murray L *et al*: DECRA Trial Investigators: Australian and New Zealand Intensive Care Society Clinical Trials Group. Decompressive craniectomy in diffuse traumatic brain injury. *N Engl J Med.* 2011;**364**:1493–502.

52. Hutchinson PJ, Kolias AG, Timofeev IS et al. RESCUEicp Trial Collaborators. Trial of decompressive craniectomy for traumatic intracranial hypertension. *N Engl J Med.* 2016;**375**:1119–30.

53. Van Essen TA, Dijkman MD, Cnossen MC, et al. Comparative effectiveness of surgery for acute subdural hematoma. *J Neurotrauma.* 2016;**33**:A-20.

54. Gregson BA, Rowan EN, Francis R, et al. STITCH (TRAUMA) Investigators. Surgical Trial In Traumatic intraCerebral Haemorrhage (STITCH): a randomised controlled trial of early surgery compared with initial conservative treatment. *Health Technol Assess.* 2015;**19**:1–138.

55. Chan AW, Tetzlaff JM, Gotzsche PC, et al. SPIRIT 2013 explanation and elaboration: guidelines for protocols of clinical trials. *BMJ* 2013;**346**:e7586.

56. Silver JM, McAllister TW, Yudofsky SC. *Textbook of Traumatic Brain Injury.* Washington DC: American Psychiatric Pub 2011.

57. Kurland D, Hong C, Aarabi B, et al. Haemorrhagic progression of a contusion after traumatic brain injury: a review. *J Neurotrauma* 2012;**29**:19–31.

58. Khoshyomn S, Tranmer BI. Diagnosis and management of paediatric closed head injury. *Semin Pediatr Surg* 2004;**13**:80–6.

59. Haaselsberger K, Pucher R, Auer LM. Prognosis after acute subdural or epidural haemorrhage. *Acta Neurochir* 1988;**90**:111–6.

60. Arciniegas D, Adler L, Topkoff J, et al. Attention and memory dysfunction after traumatic brain injury: cholinergic mechanisms, sensory gating, and a hypothesis for further investigation. *Brain Inj* 1999;**13(1)**:1–13.

61. Mathias JL, Wheaton P. Changes in attention and information-processing speed following severe traumatic brain injury: a meta-analytic review. *Neuropsychology* 2007;**21(2)**:212–23.

62. Cicerone K, Levin H, Malec J, et al. Cognitive rehabilitation interventions for executive function: moving from bench to

bedside in patients with traumatic brain injury. *J Cogn Neurosci* 2006;**18**(7):1212–22.

63. Jorge RE, Arciniegas DB. Mood disorders after TBI. *Psychiatric Clinics of North America* 2014;**37**(1):13–29.

64. Rao V, Lyketsos C. Neuropsychiatric sequelae of traumatic brain injury. *Psychosomatics* 2000;**41**(2):95–103.

65. Wood RL, Liossi C, Wood L. The impact of head injury neurobehavioural sequelae on personal relationships: preliminary findings. *Brain Injury* 2005;**19**(10):845–51.

66. Claude Blais M, Boisvert JM. Psychological and marital adjustment in couples following a traumatic brain injury (TBI): a critical review. *Brain Injury* 2005;**19**(14):1223–35.

67. Sariaslan A, Sharp DJ, D'Onofrio BM, et al. Long term outcomes associated with traumatic brain injury in childhood and adolescence: a nationwide Swedish cohort study of a wide range of medical and social outcomes. *PLoS Med* 2016;**13**(8):e1002103.

68. Radford K, Phillips J, Drummond A, et al. Return to work after traumatic brain injury: cohort comparison and economic evaluation. *Brain Inj* 2013;**27**(5):507–20.

69. Alexander MP. Mild traumatic brain injury: pathophysiology, natural history and clinical management. *Neurology* 1995;**45**:1253–60.

70. Ponsford J, Willmott C, Rothwell A, et al. Factors influencing outcome following mild traumatic brain injury in adults. *J Int Neuropsychol Soc* 2000;**6**:568–79.

71. Hou R, Moss-Morris R, Peveler R, et al. When a minor head injury results in enduring symptoms: a prospective investigation of risk factors for postconcussional syndrome after mild traumatic brain injury. *J Neurol Neurosurg Psychiatry* 2012;**83**:217–23.

72. Ryan LM, Warden DL. Post concussion syndrome. *Int Rev Psychiatry* 2003;**15**:310–16.

73. Sbordone RJ, Liter JC, Pettler-Jennings P. Recovery of function following severe traumatic brain injury: a retrospective 10-year follow-up. *Brain Inj* 1995;**9**(3):285–99.

74. Christensen BK, Colella B, Inness E, et al. Recovery of cognitive function after traumatic brain injury: a multilevel modelling analysis of Canadian outcomes. *Arch Phys Med Rehabil* 2008;**89**(12): S3–S15.

75. Cope DN, Hall, K. Head injury rehabilitation: benefit of early intervention. *Arch Phys Med Rehabil* 1982;**63**(9):433–7.

76. Powell J, Heslin J, Greenwood R. Community based rehabilitation after severe traumatic brain injury: a randomised controlled trial. *J Neurol Neurosurg Psychiatry* 2002;**72**:193–202.

77. Oddy M, da Silva Ramos S. The clinical and cost benefits of investing in neurobehavioural rehabilitation: a multi-centre study. *Brain Injury* 2013;**27**:1500–7.

78. Walker WC, Ketchum JM, Marwitz, JH, et al. A multicentre study on the clinical utility of post-traumatic amnesia duration in predicting global outcome after moderate-severe traumatic brain injury. *J Neurol Neurosurg Psychiatry* 2010;**81**(1):87–9.

79. Sigurdardottir S, Andelic N, Wehling E et al. Neuropsychological functioning in a national cohort of severe traumatic brain injury: demographic and acute injury-related predictors. *J Head Trauma Rehabil*, 2015;**30**(2):E1–12.

80. De Guise E, Leblanc J, Feyz M, et al. Effect of an integrated reality orientation programme in acute care on post-traumatic amnesia in patients with traumatic brain injury. *Brain Inj* 2005;**19**(4):263–9.

81. Thomas H, Feyz M, LeBlanc J, et al. North Star Project: reality orientation in an acute care setting for patients with traumatic brain injuries. *J Head Trauma Rehabil* 2003;**18**(3):292–302.

82. Langhorn L, Sorensen JC, Pedersen PU. A critical review of the literature on early rehabilitation of patients with

post-traumatic amnesia in acute care. *J Clin Nurs* 2010;**19(21–22)**:2959–69.

83. Cnossen, MC, Lingsma HF, Tenovuo O, et al. Rehabilitation after traumatic brain injury: A survey in 70 European neurotrauma centres participating in the CENTER-TBI study. *J Rehabil Med* 2017;**49**(5):395–401.

84. Turner-Stokes L, Disler PB, Nair A, et al. Multi-disciplinary rehabilitation for acquired brain injury in adults of working age. *Cochrane Database Syst Rev* 2005;3(3): CD004170.

85. Slade A, Tennant A, Chamberlain MA. A randomised controlled trial to determine the effect of intensity of therapy upon length of stay in a neurological rehabilitation setting. *J Rehab Med* 2002;**34(6)**:260–6.

86. Goldman SM, Kamel F, Ross GW, et al. Head injury, alpha-synuclein Rep 1, and Parkinson's Disease. *Ann Neurol* 2012;**71**:40–8.

87. Mayeux R, Ottman R, Maestre G, et al. Synergistic effects of traumatic head injury and apolipoprotein-epsilon 4 in patients with Alzheimer's Disease. *Neurology* 1995;**45(3 Pt 1)**:555–7.

88. McKee AC, Stern RA, Nowinski CJ, et al. The spectrum of disease in chronic traumatic encephalopathy. *Brain* 2013;**136**(Pt 1):43–64.

89. Roozenbeek B, Maas AIR, Menon DK. Changing patterns in the epidemiology of traumatic brain injury. *Nat Rev Neurol.* 2013;**9(4)**:231–6.

90. WHO Global status report on road safety 2015.

91. WHO, UNODC, UNDP. Global status report on violence prevention 2014.

92. Liu BC, Ivers R, Norton R, et al. Helmets for preventing injury in motorcycle riders. *Cochrane Database Syst Rev.* 2008;(1): CD004333.

93. Macpherson A, Spinks A. Bicycle helmet legislation for the uptake of helmet use and prevention of head injuries. *Cochrane Database Syst Rev.* 2008;(3):CD005401.

94. Debinski B, Clegg Smith K, Gielen A. Public opinion on motor vehicle-related injury prevention policies: a systematic review of a decade of research. *Traffic Inj Prev.* 2014;**15**:243–51.

95. Sethi M, Heidenberg J, Wall SP, et al. Bicycle helmets are highly protective against traumatic brain injury within a dense urban setting. *Injury.* 2015;**46**:2483–90.

96. Chiu WT, Kuo CY, Hung CC, et al. The effect of the Taiwan motorcycle helmet use law on head injuries. *Am J Public Health.* 2000;**90**:793–6.

97. Busko A, Hubbard Z, Zakrison T. Motorcycle-helmet laws and public health. *N Engl J Med.* 2017;**376**:1208–9.

98. Coben JH, Zhu M. Keeping an eye on distracted driving. *JAMA.* 2013;**309**:877–8.

99. Perel P, Prieto-Merino D, Shakur H, et al. Predicting early death in patients with traumatic bleeding: development and validation of prognostic model. *BMJ* 2012;**345**:e5166.

100. Health and Social Care Information Centre. Accident and emergency attendances in England—2012–2013. January 2014.

101. Obermeyer Z, Abujaber S, Maker M, et al. on behalf of the Acute Care Development Consortium. Emergency care in 59 LMICs: a systematic review. *Bull World Health Organ* 2015;**93**:577–86.

102. El Khamlichi A. Neurosurgery in Africa. *Clin Neurosurg* 2005;**52**:214–17.

103. Hartholt KA, Van Lieshout EM, Polinder S, et al. Rapid increase in hospitalizations resulting from fall-related traumatic head injury in older adults in The Netherlands 1986–2008. *J Neurotrauma* 2011;**28**:739–44.

104. Harvey LA, Close JC. Traumatic brain injury in older adults: characteristics, causes and consequences. *Injury* 2012;**43**:1821–6.

105. Murphy TE, Baker DI, Leo-Summers LS, et al. Trends in fall-related traumatic brain injury among older persons in Connecticut from 2000–2007. *J Gerontol Geriatr Res.* 2014;**3**:1000168.

106. Dams-O'Connor K, Gibbons LE, Landau A, et al. Health problems precede traumatic brain injury in older adults. *J Am Geriatr Soc* 2016;**64**:844–8.

107. Nakahara S, Ichikawa M, Kimura A. Population strategies and high-risk-individual strategies for road safety in Japan. *Health Policy* 2011;**100**:247–55.

108. Youngers EH, Zundel K, Gerhardstein D, et al. Comprehensive review of the ThinkFirst injury prevention programs: a 30-year success story for organized neurosurgery. *Neurosurgery* 2017;**81**:416–21.

109. Utomo WK, Gabbe BJ, Simpson PM, et al. Predictors of in-hospital mortality and 6-month functional outcomes in older adults after moderate to severe traumatic brain injury. *Injury* 2009;**40(9)**:973–7.

110. Mosenthal AC, Lavery RF, Addis M, et al. Isolated traumatic brain injury: age is an independent predictor of mortality and early outcome. *J Trauma* 2002;**52**(5):907–11.

111. Cremer OL, Moons KGM, van Dijk GW, et al. Prognosis following severe head injury: development and validation of a model for prediction of death, disability and functional recovery. *J Trauma* 2006;**61(6)**:1484–91.

112. Fuller GW, Kemp SP. The International Rugby Board (IRB) pitch side concussion assessment trial: a pilot test accuracy study. *Br J Sports Med* 2015;**49**:529–35.

113. McCrory P, Meeuwisse W, Dvořák J, et al. Consensus statement on concussion in sport—the 5th international conference on concussion in sport held in Berlin, October 2016. *Br J Sports Med.* 2017;**51**:838–47.

114. Harmon KG, Drezner JA, Gammons M, et al. American Medical Society for Sports Medicine position statement: concussion in sport. *Br J Sports Med.* 2013;**47**:15–26.

115. Giza CC, Kutcher JS, Ashwal S, et al. Summary of evidence-based guideline update: evaluation and management of concussion in sports: report of the Guideline Development Subcommittee of the American Academy of Neurology. *Neurology* 2013;**80**:2250–7.

116. Vagnozzi R, Tavazzi B, Signoretti S, et al. Temporal window of metabolic brain vulnerability to concussions: mitochondrial-related impairment—part I. *Neurosurgery* 2007;**61**:379–88.

117. Cantu RC. Second impact syndrome. *Clin Sports Med* 1998;**17**:37–44.

118. Bey T, Ostick B. Second impact syndrome. *West J Emerg Med.* 2009;**10**(1):6–10.

Critical Care Management of Traumatic Brain Injury

Ximena Watson and Michael Puntis

Introduction

Brain trauma includes a heterogenous group of injury patterns followed by complex, multisystem pathophysiological responses. Young adults, typically injured by high energy forces, often have concurrent extra-cranial injuries while older adults, injured following relatively low energy mechanisms, are more likely to be affected by comorbidities at the time of injury. The heterogeneity of traumatic brain injury (TBI) limits the generalisability of trial data, and the nuances of TBI management may require a knowledge-based approach rather than an evidence-based approach. A clear understanding of the pathological processes is therefore essential to providing high quality neurocritical care. Although brain trauma produces a diverse range of injuries, the Glasgow Coma Scale (GCS) can been used to stratify mild, moderate and severe TBI. A post-resuscitation GCS of 8 or less represents severe TBI. Severe TBI is typically managed in a neurosciences intensive care unit.

Pathology

The brain is usually protected from mechanical forces by the bones of the skull, the meninges and a layer of cerebrospinal fluid (CSF). However, excessive force can overwhelm these mechanisms to produce a range of focal and diffuse injury patterns. While the strength and rigidity of the skull are critical for reducing primary injury to the brain, there is a biological cost associated with mechanically protecting the brain in this way: the skull and the reflections of the dura are rigid structures and the brain is therefore enclosed within a number of non-compliant compartments. An increase in volume within any compartment, caused by haematoma or oedema, for example, is tolerated poorly. The expanding mass displaces venous blood and CSF, but when this capacity is exhausted, further increases in the intracranial volume will lead to a rapid increase in intracranial pressure (ICP). A global increase in ICP can impair cerebral perfusion while raised pressure within a localised area of brain can create a pressure gradient, which will cause shearing injury or herniation from one compartment to another.

The site and mechanism of injury has an important effect on the pattern of tissue damage, treatment options and prognosis. A direct blow to the head generally causes cerebral contusions and intracranial haemorrhage. Contusions occur when microhaemorrhages form as a consequence of damage to small blood vessels. Intra-axial haemorrhage, within the brain parenchyma, causes direct neuronal injury, but even extra-axial haemorrhage (e.g. subdural or extradural haemorrhage) can cause significant injury as a result of the mass effect.

Vehicle accidents and violent assault can cause rapid acceleration or deceleration forces which cause shearing at the interface between tissues of different density. This typically affects the grey matter/white matter junction and causes immediate axonal injury.

Penetrating injuries cause a spectrum of laceration, contusion and haemorrhage but are additionally complicated by disruption of the meninges and the introduction of foreign material with potentially infectious sequelae.

Secondary injury occurs in response to the primary event but develops beyond the injury site. Following the primary injury, a series of metabolic, inflammatory and vascular processes occur, which produce tissue damage through direct intracranial lesions, such as cerebral oedema, or haemorrhage extension. There are a number of cellular processes that lead to secondary brain injury. Excitotoxicity occurs as cell injury causes postsynaptic membranes to depolarise, leading to an uncontrolled influx of calcium ions and the release of excitatory neurotransmitters. High intracellular concentrations of calcium also activate enzymatic processes and ultimately lead to cellular death. Cellular damage also causes increased cell membrane permeability and water influx leading to cytotoxic oedema or cell rupture. Vasogenic oedema occurs as disruption of the endothelium leads to the uncontrolled transit of electrolytes and water into the extra-cellular space.

Additionally, patients with severe TBI are at risk of systemic complications, and neuronal death may occur as a result of systemic causes (e.g. hypotension, hypoxaemia or hypoglycaemia). The brain is particularly vulnerable to secondary injury due to its high metabolic demands. The oxygen requirement in the cortical grey matter is approximately $5\ ml\ 100\ ml^{-1}\ min^{-1}$, and this is usually met by very high blood flow (about 20% of cardiac output). Brain injury disrupts this balance and the supply of energy substrate falls while demand is increased. There are also complex pathophysiological changes to glucose uptake which can lead to metabolic crisis even in the presence of adequate blood flow. It is therefore important to avoid seizures and hyperthermia which increase cerebral metabolic demands, and oxygen and glucose delivery should be maintained by avoiding hypoxia, anaemia and hypoglycaemia.

Following traumatic injury, neurones and glial cells release pro-inflammatory cytokines which produce both a local and a systemic inflammatory response. Disruption of the blood–brain barrier allows these inflammatory mediators to leak into the circulation and a systemic inflammatory response is sustained. Disruption of the autonomic and neuroendocrine pathways can also cause immunosuppression, which is associated with a high rate of infective complications, such as pneumonia, and occurs commonly in TBI patients.

Immediate Management

A combination of primary and secondary injury processes will contribute to neurological damage; however, only the secondary injury is amenable to intervention and is therefore the focus of almost all current therapeutic options.

Modern trauma systems allow critical care management of TBI to be initiated rapidly by pre-hospital teams. The capabilities of the responder and the available resources may vary, but the clinical priorities remain the same. A rapid assessment needs to be performed, usually in parallel with the initial resuscitation. Life-threatening injuries need to be identified and treated, and the patient must then be transported to a trauma centre.

A number of pre-hospital interventions can reduce secondary brain injury. Tracheal intubation may be performed to control hypoxia or ventilation and to facilitate the transfer of agitated and combative patients. Haemorrhage control and the administration of fluids (including blood and blood products) can improve cerebral oxygen delivery and osmotherapy can be used to rapidly improve cerebral perfusion.

While these interventions are valuable, scene times should be minimised and urgent transfer to appropriate definitive care is essential. Despite high quality, rapid intervention many patients with severe TBI will have already sustained a secondary injury by the time they arrive in hospital. Hypotension, normally as a result of extra-cranial injuries, and hypoxia, as a result of aspiration or airway obstruction, frequently co-exist in the early stages of TBI and have been shown to be associated with increased mortality.

When the potentially brain injured patient arrives in the Emergency Department a rapid assessment needs to be made to ensure that any immediate life-threatening conditions are identified and treated. The first priority is usually to ensure the airway is patent; this may require tracheal intubation. The pharyngeal and laryngeal reflexes are frequently impaired in patients with severe TBI, and it may also be necessary to intubate the trachea to prevent aspiration of gastric contents. If the decision is made to intubate, it is important to use an appropriate technique that avoids precipitating hypotension, hypoxia or a significant increase in ICP. While intubation may be an emergency in the context of airway obstruction, there is often time to perform a focused neurological examination to determine the GCS, pupillary size and reactivity, and the presence of signs of spinal cord injury. Following the induction of anaesthesia, further clinical assessment will be limited. Cervical spine injuries need to be considered in conjunction with airway management, some injuries may be potentially unstable and there is a risk of iatrogenic spinal cord injury.[1] There is some controversy about cervical spine immobilisation, but it is important to consider the risk of cord injury particularly during intubation. Manual inline stabilisation (MILS) should be used during laryngoscopy and the use of more advanced airway techniques, such as video laryngoscopy, may help to limit the forces transmitted to the cervical spine.

Despite a general consensus on the early management goals in TBI treatment, there is little empirical evidence to support specific physiological targets, and consequently there is controversy regarding specific resuscitation endpoints. Periods of hypotension should be strenuously avoided: the current Brain Trauma Foundation guidelines recommend an initial systolic blood pressure target between 100 and 110 mmHg to maintain cerebral perfusion. Other early resuscitation priorities include maintaining normothermia and glycaemic control.

Early computed tomography (CT) imaging is necessary to identify the type and severity of the injury and resuscitation may occur in parallel with preparation for imaging.

There are very few pharmacological agents that have been proven to be beneficial in early severe TBI. A meta-analysis of randomised controlled trials of tranexamic acid in TBI suggests a reduction in haemorrhage extension and mortality; however, the data were inconsistent. The CRASH-3 trial[2] evaluated the safety and effectiveness of tranexamic acid in isolated TBI and demonstrated that early administration was associated with a reduction in the risk of death in moderate and mild head injury; however, there was no survival benefit in the severe TBI group.

Patients who have been taking anticoagulants prior to the injury and patients who are coagulopathic should have their clotting corrected to avoid haemorrhage extension. Patients who are treated with anti-platelet drugs prior to injury have worse outcomes following TBI; however, correcting platelet inhibition with platelet transfusions is not associated with improved outcomes.[3]

Critical Care Management

High quality critical care management is essential and most patients with severe TBI are cared for in a regional neuroscience intensive care unit (NICU). These specialist centres provide advanced monitoring, imaging and neurosurgical input, and they are typically associated with better outcomes.[4] However, simple measures are also important, and elevating the head of bed at 30–45°, for example, can significantly reduce ICP and improve cerebral perfusion.

Assessment

Neurological examination is an important assessment tool, even for patients who are unconscious or sedated. Deterioration may be identified by the regular assessment of the GCS and measurement of pupil diameter and reactivity to light. However, there are many factors that can make this basic assessment difficult. The motor response is the most consistently assessable component of the GCS score, and a GCS assessment may be inaccurate if tracheal intubation prevents a verbal response or facial injuries prevent eye opening.

Pupillary diameter and reactivity are important clinical signs but can be affected by a variety of mechanisms including oculomotor or optic nerve injury, localised eye injuries, and both pontine and midbrain dysfunction. The underlying injury should also be considered: an isolated unilateral third nerve palsy will not affect the consensual light reflex, while an optic nerve injury will disrupt both direct and indirect responses. Loss of the pupillary reflex is usually an indicator of more severe injury and 70–90% of patients with bilaterally unreactive pupils will have a very poor outcome.

Pupillary reaction to light can be assessed using a torch, although this is associated with poor inter-rater accuracy. Automated pupillometry uses a handheld device to measure pupil size and light reactivity with a high degree of accuracy and is especially valuable when the pupil is small.

Despite the value of bedside clinical assessment, neuroimaging is essential for diagnosis, to guide surgical interventions and for prognosis. Access to early imaging is associated with improved outcomes and fewer life-threatening complications. CT is the most commonly used imaging modality for guiding the care of TBI patients. However, normal CT appearances do not exclude a significant injury and injury patterns such as traumatic axonal injury (TAI) can be difficult to identify on CT. There may be a role for magnetic resonance imaging (MRI) in this setting; diffusion-weighted MRI can identify the microvascular shearing and microhaemorrhages associated with axonal injury. However, its use in the acute setting is limited because unstable patents with high ICP cannot tolerate the prolonged supine positioning required for MRI.

Systemic Management

Haemodynamic instability is frequently seen in patients with TBI and even brief periods of hypotension are associated with increased mortality. It is important to achieve adequate systemic blood pressure (SBP) so that the cerebral perfusion pressure is maintained. Fluid restriction is not recommended, and cardiac output monitoring should be used to adjust fluid administration to maintain euvolaemia. Vasopressors or inotropes may be required; however, catecholamines released following brain injury can induce myocardial ischaemia and impaired ventricular function, which may make it difficult to achieve SBP targets.

Table 4.1 Physiological targets for the management of severe traumatic brain injury

Ventilation	PaO_2 10–12 kPa
	$PaCO_2$ 4.5–5.0 kPa
	PEEP 5–12 mmHg
	V_T <8 ml kg^{-1} (if neuroprotective approach allows)
Cardiovascular	SBP 110 mmHg (100 mmHg if aged 50–69 years)
	MAP >90 mmHg
	Euvolaemia
	Haemoglobin 100 g l^{-1}
	Vaspressors / inotropes as required
ICP and CPP	ICP <22 mmHg
	CPP 50–70 mmHg
Biochemical	Normoglycaemia
	Serum sodium 145–155mmol l^{-1}
Other	Normothermia
	Seizure control

CPP, cerebral perfusion pressure; ICP, intracranial pressure; SBP, systolic blood pressure; MAP, mean arterial pressure; PaO_2, arterial partial pressure of carbon dioxide; PaO_2, arterial partial pressure of oxygen; PEEP, positive end-expiratory pressure; V_T, tidal volume.

TBI can also cause disruption of inhibitory cardiovascular centres in the brainstem which can lead to the phenomenon of paroxysmal sympathetic hyperactivity (PSH). This causes cycles of agitation and dystonia with pyrexia, tachycardia, hypertension and diaphoresis. Treatment options include opiates, benzodiazepines and beta adrenergic antagonists.

Patients with severe TBI usually require tracheal intubation and mechanical ventilation to protect the airway and to ensure adequate oxygen delivery and carbon dioxide clearance. Hypoxia can lead to secondary injury in the brain but hyperoxia can also be harmful; oxygen should be therefore be titrated to achieve a narrow range and a target arterial partial pressure of oxygen (PaO_2) of 10–12 kPa is usually maintained. Managing carbon dioxide clearance is often more complex; cerebral vascular tone is dependent on the partial pressure of carbon dioxide (pCO_2), and control of ventilation is therefore critically important. Hypoventilation leading to hypocapnia will induce cerebral vasoconstriction, which can result in ischaemia, while hypercapnia leads to cerebral vasodilation, an increase in intracranial blood volume and subsequent increases in the ICP. Mechanical ventilation is adjusted to achieve an optimum balance and usually a target arterial partial pressure of carbon dioxide ($PaCO_2$) range of 4.5–5.0 kPa is maintained during the acute phase of severe TBI. Hyperventilation may be used to rapidly and temporarily control acute spikes in ICP, but this should be reserved for patients at risk of imminent life-threatening complications, such as herniation of the cerebellar tonsils into the foramen magnum.

Mechanical ventilation in TBI can be challenging and a balanced approach is often required. Catecholamines released following TBI may cause neurogenic pulmonary oedema, and the high tidal volumes required for optimum $PaCO_2$ control may precipitate acute lung injury (ALI). Additionally, patients with TBI may have coexisting chest injuries and are at high risk of other pulmonary complications, such as pneumonia.

Patients with severe TBI are also at risk of gastrointestinal complications. Reduced gut motility is common, but increases in intra-abdominal pressure may lead to increased ICP and regular laxatives are important to avoid constipation. Stress ulceration is also common and early enteral feeding is recommended. Ulcer prophylaxis with a proton-pump inhibitor or H_2 antagonist is used until enteral feeding is successfully established.

Haematological, Metabolic and Endocrine Management

Acute haemorrhage in isolated TBI rarely causes significant anaemia at presentation. However, 50% of patients with severe TBI will become anaemic during the first week.[5] Anaemia is associated with worse clinical outcomes, but red cell transfusion does not appear to effectively mitigate that risk.[6] The optimum haemoglobin concentration for cerebral oxygen delivery requires a favourable balance between oxygen-carrying capacity and blood viscosity. A haemoglobin target of 100 g L^{-1} is likely to achieve optimum cerebral oxygen delivery but achieving that target through allogenic red cell transfusion is associated with risks. Few clinical studies examining the optimal transfusion strategy in TBI have been performed and are often limited by significant confounders.[7] A restrictive transfusion policy is usually implemented in general critical care patients and is likely to be safe for patients who are alert and can be reliably assessed. However, an individualised transfusion strategy is required in patients with moderate and severe TBI and a haemoglobin target of 90–100 g L^{-1} is usually more appropriate.

Disordered coagulation is common following TBI and both hypocoagulable and hyper-coagulable states can occur. Functional assays, such as thromboelastometry, may therefore be more useful than routine laboratory tests in defining clotting abnormalities. The risk of deep venous thrombus is high, and thromboprophylaxis should be initiated early; pharma-cological thromboprophylaxis is usually safe after 24 hours of clinical stability if there are no concerning signs on repeat imaging. If thromboprophylaxis is contraindicated by other injuries or an ongoing bleeding risk, then the placement of a temporary inferior vena cava filter should be considered.

Metabolic and electrolyte abnormalities are very common after TBI. Hyperglycaemia often occurs and may result in secondary brain injury. While hyperglycaemia is associated with poor neurological outcomes in TBI, intensive glycaemic control may also be harmful and therefore intermediate glucose concentrations (7.8–10.0 mmol L^{-1}) should be targeted.[8] The administration of hypotonic glucose solutions can worsen cerebral oedema and should be avoided.

Serum electrolyte disturbance, particularly dysnatraemia, is frequently seen in patients with TBI. Hyponatraemia is especially harmful because cerebral oedema is exacerbated and the seizure threshold is reduced. Hyponatraemia is usually a consequence of either cerebral salt wasting (CSW) or the syndrome of inappropriate antidiuretic hormone (SIADH). Brain injury can also disrupt the production of vasopressin and cause hypernatraemia secondary to central diabetes insipidus. Iatrogenic hypernatraemia, as a consequence of hypertonic saline solutions is common, but should be corrected gradually as an acute fall in osmolality will worsen cerebral oedema. Hypophosphataemia and hypomagnesaemia are also common and should be corrected to avoid lowering the seizure threshold.

Table 4.2 Diagnosis and management sodium disturbances in traumatic brain injury

Finding	SIADH	CSW	DI
Plasma volume	↑	↓	↓
Sodium balance	↑/↔	↓	↔
Water balance	↑	↓	↓
Serum sodium	↓	↓	↑
Serum osmolality	↓	↑/↔	↑
Urine sodium	↑	↑	↔
Urine osmolality	↑	↔/↑	↓
Management	Water restriction Demeclocycline ADH-receptor antagonists (vaptans)	Volume resuscitation Sodium replacement Fludrocortisone	Maintain euvolaemia Desmopressin

SIADH, syndrome of inappropriate antidiuretic hormone secretion; CSW, cerebral salt wasting syndrome; DI, diabetes insipidus; ADH, antidiuretic hormone.

The hypothalamic–pituitary–adrenal axis is often disrupted by brain injury, particularly by TAI, severe cerebral oedema and skull base fractures, or in older patients. Endocrine abnormalities are therefore common and secondary adrenal insufficiency occurs in many patients with severe TBI.[9] Screening for pituitary insufficiency should be considered in high risk patients or those with ongoing hyponatraemia, hypoglycaemia or a persisting requirement for vasopressors. Hydrocortisone may be necessary for refractory hypotension, and fludrocortisone may be added if hyponatraemia persists. The endocrine sequelae of TBI can be protracted and may impact on the chronic phases of rehabilitation.

Sedation

Patients with severe TBI are often sedated in the Intensive Care Unit. Primarily, sedation is used to control the cerebral metabolic rate, and to lower the ICP. Sedation is also important to facilitate mechanical ventilation and to prevent increases in ICP caused by coughing or straining. Additionally, as the patient becomes more aware, maintaining anxiolysis and analgesia becomes necessary.

Propofol is commonly used for sedation in patients with TBI. Propofol decreases the cerebral metabolic rate without causing cerebral vasodilation and an infusion can be used to effectively reduce the ICP. Its favourable pharmacokinetic properties allow it to be titrated easily, with relatively rapid wake-up when stopped. Propofol is a $GABA_A$ receptor positive allosteric modulator and $GABA_A$ receptor agonist and is therefore also effective at preventing seizures. Common side effects include negative inotropy and systemic vasodilation; propofol should therefore be used with caution in patients who are hypotensive. Patients who require high doses of propofol ($4 \text{ mg kg}^{-1} \text{ hr}^{-1}$) are also at risk of developing propofol infusion syndrome, which causes metabolic acidosis, bradycardia, renal failure and rhabdomyolysis.

Opioids, such as fentanyl, are often used concurrently with propofol to provide analgesia, to facilitate more effective mechanical ventilation and to mitigate the effects of PSH.

'Wake-up' tests to clinically assess the neurological status of patients often lead to significant deterioration and should not be performed. When a patient starts to recover, and shows increased awareness of their surroundings, drugs such as clonidine and dexmedetomidine may be used to reduce agitation and to allow other sedatives to be weaned off.

Neuroprotection

There are few specific interventions that have a clear outcome benefit in severe TBI. However, the introduction of standardised protocols is important to consistently achieve optimised physiological conditions. Neuroscience intensive care units that use systematic protocols may make clinical practice more effective and the implementation of guideline-supported practice has been associated with a significant reduction in TBI mortality. Adherence to guidelines may even be causally related to improved neurological outcomes.[10]

ICP Control

Haematoma, oedema and hydrocephalus can all cause raised ICP. Localised pressure gradients cause shearing forces and can lead to herniation between compartments. High ICP also worsens regional perfusion by reducing the cerebral perfusion pressure (CPP). Intracranial pressure greater than 20 mmHg is associated with worse outcomes but there is no high-level evidence to support the use of ICP monitoring or specific thresholds for treatment. A randomised controlled trial found no difference in outcomes after severe TBI when treatment was guided by ICP monitoring.[11] Consensus guidelines vary in their recommendations for ICP monitoring but the widely adopted Brain Trauma Foundation guidelines recommend that ICP monitoring should be used in all salvageable patients with severe TBI and CT abnormalities, or a normal CT and two of: age >40, motor posturing or hypotension (systolic blood pressure <90 mmHg).[12]

When ICP monitoring is used, a sustained ICP >20 mmHg should usually be treated; however, aggressive methods of controlling ICP are associated with risks. A proportionate, tiered approach to ICP control should be used and a combination of monitoring, clinical examination and radiological findings can be considered to guide management.

Direct ICP can be measured using intraventricular or intraparenchymal devices. Intraventricular catheters have the additional benefit of allowing therapeutic CSF drainage but there is a higher risk of bleeding and ventriculitis associated with their use. Intraparenchymal monitors are more common. The ICP value and the waveform can be used to give an indication of intracranial compliance and allow the titration of therapy to specific ICP targets. A rapidly rising ICP also provides an indication of adverse events such as haematoma expansion.

The ICP is used to derive the CPP which can be used to ensure that cerebral perfusion is maintained even in the presence of intracranial hypertension. CPP is calculated as the difference between the mean arterial pressure (MAP) and the ICP. Normal vascular function may be impaired in the injured brain and cerebral blood flow may become pressure dependant if autoregulating mechanisms become disrupted. A target CPP between 60 and 70 mmHg is recommended, but aggressive attempts to achieve a CPP above 70 mmHg should be avoided because of the risk of complications, such as ALI. A number of alternative strategies for managing CPP have been proposed; a protocol developed in Lund, Sweden, advocated lower CPP targets to limit capillary hydrostatic pressure and reduce intracranial blood volume. Initial data suggested improved outcomes, but this has not been established in larger controlled trials.

There are also more sophisticated approaches to interpreting the ICP; pressure reactivity (PRx) can be used to determine an individual's autoregulatory status and set an optimal CPP for that patient.[13] The PRx is derived by a computer system which measures the relationship between SBP and the ICP. A positive correlation between MAP and ICP suggests impaired autoregulation and increases in MAP may lead to an increase in cerebral blood volume causing increases in ICP. PRx is not universally used in neuroscience intensive care units and further evaluation of the technology will be required before it is more widely employed.

Targeted Temperature Management

The role of temperature control in patients with severe TBI needs to be considered because hypothermia reduces cerebral metabolic oxygen consumption while pyrexia is associated with increased neuronal injury. Induced hypothermia has therefore been proposed both as a prophylactic method of reducing secondary brain injury and as therapeutic intervention to control intracranial hypertension.

Systemic hypothermia is associated with complications, such as infection and coagulopathy, which may outweigh any neuroprotective effects. Prophylactic hypothermia does not improve outcomes compared with normothermia,[14] but the role of therapeutic hypothermia to control ICP is more controversial. Meta-analyses have revealed inconsistent findings and post-hoc analyses suggest that patients who underwent evacuation of intracranial haematomas experienced improved outcomes when treated with early hypothermia.[15, 16] However, large randomised trials have not demonstrated a clear benefit for patients with intracranial hypertension who were cooled to 32–35°C as part of a tiered ICP control strategy.[17, 18]

Mild hypothermia at 35°C may still be a useful intervention as part of a tiered approach to lower ICP, and targeted temperature management to avoid pyrexia remains an important element of the care of TBI patients.

Osmotherapy

In patients who have early signs of raised ICP, hyperosmolar solutions can be administered to minimise cerebral oedema; using an osmotic gradient to draw extravascular water into the intravascular space. The use of hypertonic saline has become increasingly common, particularly for patients with polytrauma and haemodynamic instability. Hypertonic saline is effective at controlling ICP in addition to expanding the intravascular volume and avoiding diuresis which can lead to hypotension. Various concentrations are available and repeated doses can be administered, titrated to the serum sodium concentration. Mannitol is effective at reducing ICP at doses of $0.25–1$ g.kg^{-1} body weight and is usually administered as a 10% or 20% solution. However, increases in serum osmolality to more than 320 mOsm l^{-1} can cause neurological and renal complications and should be avoided. A number of meta-analyses have suggested that hypertonic saline may be more effective than mannitol for the treatment of intracranial hypertension.[19]

Seizure Control

Post-traumatic seizures (PTS) are a common phenomenon after severe TBI and may be under-recognised. Seizure activity leads to increases in ICP by increasing cerebral metabolic rate and, if untreated, can result in worse outcomes. Seizures that are clinically obvious should therefore be aggressively treated. Non-convulsive seizures (NCS) are harder to recognise and continuous EEG is a valuable tool in diagnosing NCS and ensuring adequate pharmacological control. Cortical spreading depolarisation can also be detected on scalp EEG and is an indicator or severe injury and poor prognosis.

Immediate seizures (less than 24 hours post-injury) occur as the impact of the injury stimulates brain tissue that has a low seizure threshold. Early seizures (occurring within 7 days) are a direct result of the injury. Secondary processes, such as the disruption of the blood–brain barrier or the unregulated release of excitatory neurotransmitters, increases the risk of seizures, and tissue disruption caused by intracranial haemorrhage or cerebral contusions may result in epileptogenesis.

Late seizures (occurring after 7 days) relate to permanent structural changes in the brain. Prophylactic anti-epileptic drugs may be used to decrease the incidence of early PTS, but this has not shown to be associated with improved outcomes.

Surgical Intervention

Although many patients with severe TBI can be managed nonsurgically, there is a critical role for surgery both in the primary evacuation of focal haematoma, and in the management of raised ICP from more diffuse injuries.

An external ventricular drain may be inserted to remove CSF; even in the absence of significant hydrocephalus, drainage of a small volume of fluid can lower the ICP in patients with reduced intracranial compliance. However, there are risks associated with the procedure and it is not routinely used.

An intracranial haematoma may be evacuated to reduce the ICP and limit further secondary injury; during haematoma evacuation, a primary decompressive craniectomy may also be performed by not replacing the craniotomy bone flap. This increases the intracranial compliance and reduces the ICP. A secondary decompressive craniectomy involves the removal of a large area of the skull vault and opening of the dura as an invasive intervention to reduce ICP. This is performed as a lifesaving intervention, although its effects on quality of life are less clear. The difficult decision to operate needs to be carefully considered by the clinical team. An individualised decision needs to be made, weighing the benefit of reduced mortality against the increased risk of severe disability.[20]

Pharmacological Management

There have been a number of therapies which initially appeared to be promising, but when phase three trials have been conducted, ultimately a clear clinical benefit has not been demonstrated. In preclinical and small clinical trials progesterone was associated with positive effects; however, larger phase 3 trials did not confirm improved outcomes. Erythropoetin (EPO) has nonhaemopoietic mechanisms which may be beneficial for endothelial cells, neurons, and glia but again, large RCTs have not demonstrated improved neurological outcome.

Animal models suggested that neuronal degeneration can be reduced by inhibiting lipid peroxidation with high doses of methylprednisolone; however, phase three trials demonstrated higher mortality in the group allocated to methylprednisone compared to placebo. Despite this, there may potentially be a role for lower dose dexamethasone which could reduce the cytogenic oedema associated with focal haemorrhage.

Neuromonitoring

Advances in multimodality neuromonitoring have allowed clinicians to move towards a more individualised approach. The aim of neuromonitoring in TBI is to evaluate the extracellular milieu in potentially viable brain so that timely intervention can be used to minimise secondary injury. Monitoring devices can use both invasive and noninvasive methods.

Brain tissue oxygen ($PbtO_2$) can be measured using intraparenchymal probes and provides an assessment of the balance between oxygen delivery and consumption. Low $PbtO_2$ is associated with worse outcomes and strategies to improve brain $PbtO_2$ have been developed. Increases in brain oxygenation can usually be achieved either by increasing cerebral blood flow or by increasing the arterial oxygen content.

Noninvasive monitoring of tissue oxygen is also possible; near infrared spectroscopy (NIRS) is a continuous direct monitor of cerebral oxygenation which acts by estimating the haemoglobin oxygen saturation of brain tissue. Its application in adult TBI is not widespread, although it has the potential to become a useful monitoring adjunct in the critical care environment. The main limitation currently is the potential for signal contamination from extra-cranial tissue. With current technology, the baseline reading for cerebral tissue regional oxygen saturation (rSO_2) can be highly variable and monitoring trends is therefore more useful. Further developments will be required before NIRS could be used as an alternative to more invasive monitoring.

Global cerebral oxygen extraction can also be measured; the jugular venous oxygen saturation ($SjvO_2$) reflects the ratio between cerebral blood flow and oxygen uptake. Jugular venous desaturation is associated with worse outcomes, but there is no evidence to indicate that targeting $SjvO_2$ is associated with improved outcomes after TBI.

Cerebral microdialysis can be used to directly evaluate localised brain metabolism.[21] A fine catheter is inserted into perilesional tissue and small-molecular-weight molecules can then be continuously or intermittently sampled from the interstitial space. The microdialysis probe is slowly and continuously perfused and the dialysate is collected and analysed. Many different assays are available although the most commonly used include brain tissue glucose, lactate and pyruvate. The lactate:pyruvate ratio (LPR) can also be calculated. An LPR of more than 25 is abnormal and values greater than 40 indicate a brain energy crisis.

In recent years there has been increasing interest in the use of systemic biomarkers to inform clinicians about both the diagnosis and prognosis in TBI. The main indication for their use to date has been in the diagnosis of mild TBI and assessment of the requirement for neuroimaging. There is also a potential role for their use in patients with polytrauma who require deep sedation when the initial CT scan does not clearly identify an anatomical lesion to demonstrate TBI. Increases in levels of blood protein biomarkers could be a helpful guide to repeat imaging or monitor ICP. Although many protein biomarkers exist, the most promising ones are S100-B, glial fibrillary acidic protein (GFAP) and neuron specific enolase, all of which have been shown to correlate with secondary injury. The significant

Table 4.3 Neuromonitoring in traumatic brain injury

Monitor	Measured variable	Invasiveness	Indications	Advantages	Disadvantages
Intraparenchymal or subdural pressure sensor	ICP PRx	Invasive	Targeted ICP control Maintenance of target CPP CPP optimisation (PRx)	Relatively easy insertion Low complication rate	Risk of bleeding and infection Measures localised pressure Zero-drift over time
External ventricular drain	ICP	Invasive	Therapeutic drainage of CSF Targeted ICP control Maintenance of target CPP CPP optimisation (PRx)	Measures global ICP Therapeutic drainage of CSF	More complex insertion Increased risk of procedural complications Risk of catheter-related ventriculitis
Brain tissue pO_2	$PbtO_2$	Invasive	Assessment of balance between oxygen delivery and metabolism	Regional assessment Continuous Defined ischaemic 'thresholds'	Risk of bleeding and infection Measures oxygenation within small region of brain
Near infrared spectroscopy	rSO_2	Noninvasive	Assessment of adequacy of cerebral oxygen delivery	Real time Measurement of multiple areas	Ischaemic threshold poorly defined. Signal contamination by extracranial tissue Limited evidence base
EEG	Seizures Disease-specific patterns SDs (possibly)	Noninvasive	Detect seizures prognostication Titration of sedative drugs	Detection of nonconvulsive seizures	Skilled interpretation required Diagnosis affected by sedative drugs

Cerebral microdialysis	Invasive	Glucose Lactate Pyruvate LPR Novel biomarkers (research purposes)	Detection of cerebral hypoxia/ischaemia Detection of cellular energy failure ICP and CPP optimisation	Assessment of cerebral metabolism, including non-ischaemic causes of metabolic dysfunction	Local measurement only Not continuous
Transcranial Doppler	Noninvasive	Blood flow velocity Pulsatility index Autoregulatory indices	Detection of cerebral hypoperfusion	Can be used for frequent measurement	Labour intensive Operator dependent Failure if no acoustic window Limited evidence base in TBI

CBF, cerebral blood flow; CPP, cerebral perfusion pressure; EEG, electroencephalography; ICP, intracranial pressure; LPR, lactate to pyruvate ratio; PRx, pressure reactivity index; PbtO$_2$, Brain tissue oxygen partial pressure; rSO$_2$, regional oxygen saturation; SD, Spreading depolarisations; TBI, traumatic brain injury.

clinical pitfall, however, is that these biomarkers only appear to increase in response to a secondary injury and not prior to the developing insult. Increases in tumour necrosis factor (TNF), interleukin-8 (IL-8) and complement factors may rise before a secondary insult has occurred thereby providing time to mitigate the risk. However, their role in diagnosis and aiding therapy has yet to be fully elucidated.

Conclusions

TBI is defined by variable degrees of primary and secondary injury and these processes often consist as a continuum. The primary injury describes irreversible structural tissue damage caused at the time of trauma and strategies to reduce the primary injury are generally limited to preventative and public health measures. Secondary injury can be modified by a range of critical care interventions. Although the evidence base for the management of TBI is incomplete, internationally endorsed guidelines exist which provide clinicians with a coherent evaluation of both empirical evidence and expert opinion. Although many specific experimental therapies have not been proven to be beneficial, meticulous and rational critical care medicine and nursing care remain important for achieving optimal clinical outcomes.

References

1. Sundheim SM, Cruz M. The evidence for spinal immobilization: an estimate of the magnitude of the treatment benefit. *Ann Emerg Med* 2006;48:217–8; author reply 18–9.

2. CRASH_Trial_Collaborators. Effects of tranexamic acid on death, disability, vascular occlusive events and other morbidities in patients with acute traumatic brain injury (CRASH-3): a randomised, placebo-controlled trial. *Lancet* 2019; 394:1713–23.

3. Holzmacher JL, Reynolds C, Patel M, et al. Platelet transfusion does not improve outcomes in patients with brain injury on antiplatelet therapy. *Brain Inj* 2018;32:325–30.

4. Dunn MS, Beck B, Simpson PM, et al. Comparing the outcomes of isolated, serious traumatic brain injury in older adults managed at major trauma centres and neurosurgical services: A registry-based cohort study. *Injury* 2019;50:1534–9.

5. Faul M, Coronado V. Epidemiology of traumatic brain injury. *Handb Clin Neurol* 2015;127:3–13.

6. Zhang W, Du K, Chen X. Benefits of red blood cell transfusion in patients with traumatic brain injury. *Crit Care* 2019;23:218.

7. Lelubre C, Bouzat P, Crippa IA, et al. Anemia management after acute brain injury. *Crit Care* 2016;20:152.

8. Kramer AH, Roberts DJ, Zygun DA. Optimal glycemic control in neurocritical care patients: a systematic review and meta-analysis. *Crit Care* 2012;16:R203.

9. Kleindienst A, Brabant G, Bock C, et al. Neuroendocrine function following traumatic brain injury and subsequent intensive care treatment: a prospective longitudinal evaluation. *J Neurotrauma* 2009;26:1435–46.

10. Gerber LM, Chiu YL, Carney N, et al. Marked reduction in mortality in patients with severe traumatic brain injury. *J Neurosurg* 2013;119(6):1583–90.

11. Chesnut RM, Temkin N, Carney N, et al. A trial of intracranial-pressure monitoring in traumatic brain injury. *N Engl J Med* 2012;367(26):2471–81.

12. Carney N, Totten AM, O'Reilly C, et al. Guidelines for the Management of Severe Traumatic Brain Injury, Fourth Edition. *Neurosurgery* 2017;80(1):6–15.

13. Depreitere B, Guiza F, Van den Berghe G, et al. Pressure autoregulation monitoring and cerebral perfusion pressure target

recommendation in patients with severe traumatic brain injury based on minute-by-minute monitoring data. *J Neurosurg* 2014;120(6):1451–7.

14. Cooper DJ, Nichol AD, Bailey M, et al. Effect of early sustained prophylactic hypothermia on neurologic outcomes among patients with severe traumatic brain injury: The POLAR randomized clinical trial. *JAMA* 2018;320(21):2211–20.

15. Clifton GL, Coffey CS, Fourwinds S, et al. Early induction of hypothermia for evacuated intracranial hematomas: a post hoc analysis of two clinical trials. *J Neurosurg* 2012;117(4):714–20.

16. Suehiro E, Koizumi H, Fujisawa H, et al. Diverse effects of hypothermia therapy in patients with severe traumatic brain injury based on the computed tomography classification of the traumatic coma data bank. *J Neurotrauma* 2015;32(5):353–8.

17. Andrews PJ, Sinclair HL, Rodriguez A, et al. Hypothermia for intracranial hypertension after traumatic brain injury. *N Engl J Med* 2015;373(25):2403–12.

18. Maekawa T, Yamashita S, Nagao S, et al. Prolonged mild therapeutic hypothermia versus fever control with tight hemodynamic monitoring and slow rewarming in patients with severe traumatic brain injury: a randomized controlled trial. *J Neurotrauma* 2015;32 (7):422–9.

19. Burgess S, Abu-Laban RB, Slavik RS, et al. A systematic review of randomized controlled trials comparing hypertonic sodium solutions and mannitol for traumatic brain injury: implications for emergency department management. *Ann Pharmacother* 2016;50(4):291–300.

20. Honeybul S, Ho KM, Lind CRP, et al. The current role of decompressive craniectomy for severe traumatic brain injury. *J Clin Neurosci* 2017;43:11–15.

21. Carteron L, Bouzat P, Oddo M. Cerebral microdialysis monitoring to improve individualized neurointensive care therapy: An update of recent clinical data. *Front Neurol* 2017;8:601.

Post-traumatic Epilepsy in Children

Cristina Rosado Coelho and Jun T. Park

Introduction

In 2014, about 2.87 million traumatic brain injury (TBI)-related emergency department (ED) visits, hospitalizations and deaths occurred in the United States. This number has increased by 53% from 2006 (approximately 1.88 million) to 2014. It has been estimated that in 2014, over 837,000 TBI-related ED visits, hospitalizations and deaths occurred among children.[1]

In addition to being an important cause of death, TBI is a common source of morbidity in children. Post-traumatic seizures (PTS), post-traumatic epilepsy (PTE) and neuropsychiatric sequelae contribute to the medical health burden that children frequently have after TBI. PTS are commonly defined by many researchers as immediate seizures (occurring less than 24 hours after TBI), early PTS (occur less than 1 week after injury) and late PTS (occur more than 1 week after TBI). PTE is usually defined as the patient having had two or more unprovoked seizures (some authors require one unprovoked seizure) following TBI.[2, 3] This chapter will be devoted to the discussion of PTE.

Epidemiology and Risk Factors

The incidence and prevalence of PTE in children is difficult to ascertain due to differences in definitions used, severity of injury and follow-up duration. Different studies show that 10–20% of children have PTE following severe TBI.[4–9] The prevalence of PTE in children ranges from 0.2% to 11%.[2, 7, 8, 10, 11] Distinct risk factors have been demonstrated to be associated with higher incidence of PTS or PTE. These risk factors are detailed in Table 5.1. Risk factors for developing PTE are: early PTS, higher severity of TBI (i.e., worse Glasgow Coma Scale (GCS)), young age, abnormal neuroimaging (subdural hematomas, uncal herniation, brain contusion, skull fractures) and/or prolonged loss of consciousness. Note, however, that some of the population studies included both children and adults without distinction between these two groups. Additionally, younger age, nonaccidental head trauma and presence of intra-axial blood were clinical predictors of subclinical seizures or status epilepticus in a prospective study that included patients who were admitted to the pediatric intensive care unit (PICU).[5] Furthermore, it is important to mention that PTE may develop 10 years after a severe TBI.[10, 11]

Pathophysiology

The pathophysiology of a TBI is poorly understood and it seems to differ significantly between a pediatric and an adult patient. It is well known that the immature brain has a higher capacity for plasticity, essential in synaptic formation. This can be an advantage as

Table 5.1 Relationship of Risk Factors and the Development of PTS or PTE in Subjects with TBI[a]

Study (design)	No. of subjects (age)	Incidence rate	Risk factors for developing immediate or early PTS	Risk factors for developing PTE
		Pediatric cohort		
Lewis et al. (1993), USA (retrospective hospital chart review)[35]	194 children (3 months–15 years)	Immediate PTS: 7% (14/194)	GCS on admission ≤ 8.	NA
Hahn et al. (1988), USA (retrospective hospital chart review and prospective follow-up between 7 months and 6 years)[8]	937 children (birth–16 years)	Immediate PTS: 9% (87/937); Early PTS: 0.3% (3/937); PTE: 0.2% (2/937)	GCS on admission ≤ 8; Diffuse cerebral edema; Acute subdural hematoma.	
Appleton and Demellweek (2002), U.K. (retrospective hospital chart review and prospective follow up of children admitted in a rehabilitation unit)[9]	102 children (1.3–15.2 years)	PTE: 9% (9/102)	NA	Early PTS; GCS on admission < 8 (marginal significance).
Emanuelson and Uvebrant (2009), Sweden (Population-based retrospective follow-up of 10 years)[7]	109 children with TBI (0–17 years)	Immediate PTS: 7% (8/109); PTE: 11% (12/109).	NA	Immediate PTS.

Table 5.1 (cont.)

Study (design)	No. of subjects (age)	Incidence rate	Risk factors for developing immediate or early PTS	Risk factors for developing PTE
Arango et al. (2012), USA (retrospective hospital chart review)[6]	130 children with severe TBI (0–17 years)	Early PTS (clinical or subclinical): 19% (25/130); PTE: 17% (22/130)	Young age (<1 year); Nonaccidental trauma; Epidural hematomas.	Presence of immediate or early PTS; Young age (<3 years); Subdural hematomas and uncal herniation.
Arndt et al. (2013), USA (Prospective in-hospital, cEEG in PICU)[5]	87 children with TBI (1 month–18 years)	Immediate or early PTS (clinical and subclinical): 44% (37/87); Status epilepticus: 18% (16/87)	Young age (< 1 year); Nonaccidental trauma; Presence of fracture on computerized tomography.	NA
Park and Chugani (2015), USA (retrospective hospital chart review)[4]	321 children with severe TBI (0–15 years)	PTE: 15% (47/321)	NA	Severe TBI.
O'Neill et al. (2015), USA (Prospective in-hospital, cEEG)[32]	144 children with TBI (0–17 years)	Immediate or early PTS (clinical and subclinical): 30% (43/144) Status epilepticus: 16%	Young age (< 2.4 years); Nonaccidental trauma.	NA
Adult and pediatric cohort				
Annegers et al. (1998 and 2000), USA	4541 children and adults (age not specified)	Immediate and early PTS: 2.6% (117/4541); PTE: 2.1% (97/4541)	NA	Brain contusion; Subdural hematoma; Severe head injuries;

Study	Study population	PTS/PTE incidence	Risk factors	Risk factors
(retrospective hospital chart review)[2]				Skull fractures; Prolonged loss of consciousness; Early PTS.
Aiskainen et al. (1999),[46] Finland (patients referred to a rehabilitation and employment program after TBI, retrospective review hospital chart and prospective follow-up ≥ 5 years)	490 children and adult (0.8–71 years): 241 subjects ≤ 16 years of age	Subjects ≤ 16 years of age: Early PTS: 24% (59/241); PTE: 30% (74/241)	Young age (< 7 years)	Early PTS; Depressed skull fracture; Young age.
Thapa et al. (2010), India (Prospective observation hospital study)[41]	520 adults and children (14 days–89 years); 93 subjects ≤10 years of age	Subjects ≤10 years of age: Immediate PTS: 11% (10/93) Early PTS: 4% (4/93) PTE: 3% (3/93)	Both children and adult: TBI due to fall from height Associated medical problems (hypertension, diabetes mellitus, chronic airway disorders, liver diseases, cerebrovascular disease and renal failure at the time of injury); Severity of TBI.	
Zhao et al. (2012),[47] China (retrospective hospital follow-up)	2826 adults and children (4–79 years of age): 288 subjects ≤ 19 years of age	Subjects ≤ 19 years of age: PTE: 4% (12/288)	NA	Both children and adult: Older patients (particularly > 50 years of age); Severity of TBI; Higher number of surgery interventions;

Table 5.1 (cont.)

Study (design)	No. of subjects (age)	Incidence rate	Risk factors for developing immediate or early PTS	Risk factors for developing PTE
Wang et al. (2013),[48] China (retrospective hospital chart review)	3093 adults and children (1 month–95 years old): 320 subjects ≤14 years of age	Subjects ≤14 years of age: PTS 11% (34/320) (not specified timing of PTS)	Both children and adult: Frontal-temporal lobar contusion; Linear fracture; Severity of TBI.	Contusions; Intraparenchymal brain hemorrhages; Early PTS.

[a]It was not possible to specify the risk factors for immediate/early PTS vs. PTE for some studies because the authors did not make that distinction.

cEEG, continuous electroencephalography; GCS, Glasgow Coma Scale; NA, Not available; PICU, Pediatric intensive care unit; PTE, post-traumatic epilepsy; PTS, post-traumatic seizures; TBI, Traumatic brain injury an injury in the developing brain may activate undefined mechanisms responsible for architectural and functional modifications of neuronal networks, maximizing the functional outcome.[12] However, plasticity in a maturing brain can also be a source of vulnerability due to early imbalances in excitatory/inhibitory transmission. The proposed mechanisms to support this finding are postsynaptic decrease in $GABA_A$ receptor sensitivity and/or expression, changes in the ratio between postsynaptic expression of $GABA_A$/$GABA_B$ receptors and decrease in presynaptic inhibitory interneuron activity.[12] Additionally, mechanisms involved in epileptogenesis may include alterations in GABA-receptor-mediated postsynaptic inhibition, with the post-TBI-induced seizures occurring in part due to the reduction of $GABA_A$-mediated inhibition.[12] Other possible contributing factors associated with age-dependent differences include: lower expression of the glutamate type 1 receptor (with a slower clearance from the synaptic cleft) and N-methyl-d-aspartate (NMDA) receptors that are more permeable to Ca^{2+} with slower desensitization, thereby increasing excitability in the developing brain.[13]

Neuroinflammation may also play a role in the development of PTE. After a TBI, there is a cerebral inflammatory response which includes blood–brain barrier (BBB) dysfunction, edema, microglial, astrocytic activation and migration, and the release of inflammatory factors. The inflammatory factors include cytokines (including tumor necrosis factor (TNF-α), transforming growth factor-β (TGF-β) and interleukin-1β (IL-1β), -6 and -10, with downstream activation of intracellular signaling cascades involving nuclear factor Kappa light-chain-enhancer of activated B cells (NF-κB) and the resultant recruitment of blood-derived leukocytes into brain parenchyma. Although important in promoting tissue repair, microglia and astrocytes promote inflammation with production of cytotoxic factors and cytokines. All of the above contribute to edema, oxidative stress, the production of more cytokines and neurotoxic proteases, propagating the inflammatory cascade.[13]

Additionally, increasing evidence suggests that neuroinflammation (with activation of microglia and production of proinflammatory cytokines) may be a common consequence of epileptic seizure activity.[14] Analysis of cerebrospinal fluid (CSF) from newly diagnosed adult patients with tonic-clonic seizures detected an upregulation of IL-6 and IL-1 receptors (IL-1Rs). Matched serum samples revealed higher levels of IL-6 in the CSF, suggesting that these cytokines likely originated in the brain. High levels of cytokines including IL-1β and high-mobility group box protein-1 (HMGB1) have also been identified in neurons and glia of surgically resected epileptic tissue.[15–17] Conversely, the demonstration that glial cell activation and recruitment, and the synthesis of inflammatory factors may precede and/or occur concurrently with epileptogenic events support the hypothesis that neuroinflammation may also contribute to epileptogenicity after TBI. Interactions between neurons, glia and inflammatory mediators (HMGB1 interacting with toll-like receptors, IL-1β interacting with its receptors and TGF-β signaling from extravascular albumin in an immature brain) have all been implicated in promoting seizure susceptibility.[13]

Lastly, age-dependent differences in seizure susceptibility and neuroinflammation may contribute to a heightened vulnerability to epileptogenesis in young patients with TBI in comparison to adult patients. There is a higher upregulation of chemokines, higher levels of cytokines (IL-1α, IL-6, IL-12 and TNF-α) in CSF and serum, and differences in the activation of microglia, macrophages and neutrophil infiltration.[13] Although these findings have been seen in multiple studies with different models, the mechanisms underlying the relationship between the inflammatory environment, age-dependent differences and epileptogenesis, particularly in the context of brain injury, remain poorly understood.

Furthermore, different biomarkers seem to be associated with PTE. Genetic association studies have suggested various predisposing genetic traits contributing to the development of PTE: single nucleotide polymorphism (SNP) rs1143634 of interleukin-1β (IL-1β) gene, SNPs rs3791878 and rs769391 of the glutamic acid decarboxylase 1 (GAD1) gene, SNPs rs3766553 and rs10920573 of the adenosine A1 receptor (A1AR) gene and the functional variant C677T of the methylenetetrahydrofolate reductase (MTHFR) enzyme.[18] The most noteworthy biomarkers identified were IL-1β rs1143634 and A1AR rs10920573. Both had heterogenous at-risk genotypes (Cytosine-Thymine (CT)). Those with IL-1β rs1143634 CT genotype developed PTE in 47.7% of cases (p = 0.008) and this CT genotype was also associated with lower IL-1β serum levels and a higher CSF/serum IL-1β ratio. The IL-1β rs1143634 TT genotype was suggested to be protective.[19] Those with A1AR rs10920573 CT genotype developed PTE in 19.2% of cases (p = 0.022).[20] However, limitations of these genetic association studies included small sample sizes and some heterogeneity regarding the definition of PTS versus PTE.

Additionally, brain-derived peripheral biomarkers have been studied after TBI, particularly the glial protein S100B. TBI is associated with a rapid loss of BBB integrity followed (or in the absence) by brain injury. The S100B is a candidate peripheral biomarker of BBB permeability, reflecting the presence of BBB disruption and may have a role in predicting or ruling out brain injury. Due to the fact that serious intracranial events are associated with an increased risk for seizures, S100B may also prove useful in the future in detecting individuals at low risk versus those who will likely develop posttraumatic sequelae. Nonetheless, the correct interpretation of blood biomarkers related to the central nervous system (CNS) can be challenging, as most of these biomarkers are expressed to varying degrees outside the CNS.[21, 22]

Finally, neurophysiologic biomarkers can also be considered. Angeleri and collaborators followed prospectively 137 patients aged between 15 and 65 years for 12 months after TBI. They demonstrated that the presence of focal electroencephalography (EEG) abnormalities (focal slow and/or epileptiform activity) detected at 1 month after TBI was associated with a 3.49 fold increased risk of PTE 95% confidence interval, CI: 1.10–11.05, adjusting for low GCS scores, early seizures and single focal lesions on brain computerized tomography.[23] A more recent study by Kim and collaborators performed a retrospective case–control study of risk factors for PTE, in which 25 consecutive patients who developed epilepsy within 1 year of a TBI were matched by injury severity and age to 25 controls who did not develop epilepsy within 1 year of the trauma, for patients aged ≥ 18 years. Epileptiform abnormalities in EEG (i.e., seizures, sporadic epileptiform discharges, lateralized or generalized periodic discharges and lateralized rhythmic delta activity) were associated with PTE (odds ratio, OR: 3.5 95% CI: 0.99–11.68, p=0.042). When evaluating individual subtypes of EEG epileptiform abnormalities, only sporadic epileptiform discharges were associated with PTE (OR: 4.57 95% CI: 1.60–21, p=0.007). These findings remained significant even after controlling for subdural hematoma (another independent factor that was shown to contribute to increased risk for PTE in this study). Differences in sporadic epileptiform discharges between cases and controls were already apparent within 5 days of the head trauma. The authors suggested that early EEG could be a useful diagnostic tool to assess TBI patients for PTE risk. Interestingly, EEG focal polymorphic slowing was also found to be associated with PTE on univariate analysis (OR: 2.67 95% CI: 0.97–10.1, p=0.04).[24]

Clinical Presentation

TBI in the pediatric population is associated with a high mortality rate and long-term morbidities, including motor, cognitive, behavioral and language impairments. As previously mentioned, another important consequence is the development of PTS and PTE.

Although the initial seizure type may be difficult to lateralize (due to TBI severity involving multifocal regions in the brain), some studies in pediatric patients have shown that focal seizure activity is the most common seizure type followed by generalized tonic-clonic activity.[25] Infants can have focal seizures presenting with generalized seizure semiology, as in symmetric/asymmetric epileptic spasms or generalized tonic seizures.[25] In a retrospective study of pediatric patients diagnosed with PTE, about 19% of patients (6 out of 31) had epileptic spasms.[4] Furthermore, a higher severity of TBI is associated with multiple seizure types.[4, 26] PTE can occur as late as 10 years after TBI. However, in the majority of patients (75%), the onset is within the first year after TBI.[7, 10]

After a TBI, there is an increased risk of psychiatric diagnosis, including depression, anxiety, posttraumatic stress disorder, obsessive-compulsive disorder, panic disorder and attention deficit hyperactivity disorder. Various episodic nonepileptic phenomena, mainly of psychopathologic nature or misinterpreted behavior, are characterized by paroxysmal movements, unusual sensations and staring. The presence of these nonepileptic events in a patient make the diagnosis of seizures more challenging.[27]

Assessment and Diagnosis

Head computerized tomography is the recommended neuroimaging in the acute setting after a severe TBI. Various abnormalities can be found, including fracture, hemorrhage, contusion, pneumocephalus, edema, herniation and compressed basal cisterns.[28, 29] In the management of pediatric severe TBI, routinely obtaining a repeat computerized tomography scan >24 hours after the admission and initial follow-up are not suggested for making decisions about neurosurgical intervention, unless there is either evidence of neurologic deterioration or increasing ICP.[30]

Brain magnetic resonance imaging (MRI) is the study of choice, particularly for non-acute evaluations of PTE, providing the highest sensitivity to detect structural brain changes. Fluid attenuated inversion recovery (FLAIR) is helpful in detecting contusion, diffuse axonal injury, blood, edema or encephalomalacia. Other sequences are also helpful in detecting microhemorrhages, such as gradient echo (GRE) or susceptibility-weighted imaging (SWI). However, it is important to mention that some features can be transiently found in FLAIR or diffusion-weighted imaging (DWI) sequences after repeated and prolonged seizures.[31]

The utility of continuous electroencephalography (cEEG) has been studied in pediatric patients admitted to the hospital due to an acute mild to severe TBI. These studies showed that 7% to 16% of patients with TBI had only subclinical seizures and status epilepticus was identified in 11% to 18%. The incidence of status epilepticus in mild TBI was 12%, moderate TBI was 11% and severe TBI was 31%. Between 30% and 40% of patients had clinical or subclinical seizures.[5, 32] Although there is no clear evidence that the routine use of cEEG can change the outcome, some potential benefits can be described including assistance in establishing the correct differential diagnosis and adequate treatment, avoidance of treatment of nonepileptic events and eventually some assistance with prognosis.[33] These advantages propose a role for EEG monitoring to detect seizures in children with TBI in the acute setting, particularly in severe TBI.[32, 34] In a patient presenting with a possible first epileptic seizure months or years after the TBI, a 10-20 system EEG can be helpful in the differential diagnosis. An interictal EEG showing epileptiform discharges has a specificity of >97% for epilepsy, despite a low sensitivity of 30–50%. A video-EEG monitoring also has a role in clarifying differential diagnosis and localizing the suspected epileptogenic zone.[31]

Management

The most recent guidelines for the management of severe TBI in children recommends that prophylactic antiepileptic drug (AED) therapy may be considered to reduce the incidence of clinical or subclinical early PTS (within 7 days).[30] This recommendation was supported by a single center retrospective cohort study of children between ages 3 months and 15 years. Lewis and collaborators reported a significant reduction in early PTS rate in patients after a severe TBI, treated with prophylactic phenytoin compared with those not treated prophylactically (15% vs. 53%, p-value = 0.04).[35] These results are in alignment with those of Temkin and collaborators. They performed a prospective double-blind and placebo-controlled study to determine the effect of treatment with phenytoin on early and late PTS in 404 adult patients. In the treated group, the incidence of early PTS was 3.6% (p-value < 0.001) compared with placebo (14.2%) (risk ratio, 0.27; 95% confidence interval CI, 0.12–0.62). Treatment with phenytoin had no effect on either late PTS or survival compared with placebo with a follow-up of up to 2 years.[36] These findings are not seen uniformly in all studies with some authors reporting no statistically significant difference in rates of early PTS between phenytoin and placebo.[37, 38]

A few studies tried to understand which AED would be better for the treatment of pediatric patients with TBI. Pearl and collaborators demonstrated feasibility and tolerability of levetiracetam in the context of epilepsy prevention following TBI in a high-risk pediatric population (defined as intracranial hemorrhage or penetrating injury, depressed skull fracture with subdural hemorrhage or early PTS). Forty-five patients aged between 6 and 7 years were recruited and followed up for 2 years. Twenty children were treated with levetiracetam 55 mg/Kg/day, for 30 days, starting within 8 hours post-TBI. This study showed a high compliance (95%), no higher incidence of infection, mood changes or behavior problems among treatment and observational subjects. Only 1 (2.5%) of 40 patients developed PTE.[39] However, a recent prospective study analyzed the prevalence of early PTS in children who were admitted to the PICU and placed on levetiracetam as a seizure prophylaxis after a moderate to severe TBI. The percentage of children who develop early clinical PTS while on levetiracetam (17.6%) is similar to that reported in the literature for children who do not receive seizure prophylaxis (20–53%). In comparison, the percentage of children who develop early PTS while receiving phenytoin is lower (2–15%).[26, 35, 40, 41] Nevertheless, since these were not comparative studies the significance of these results should be interpreted cautiously. Additionally, other clinical factors (such as sample size, different types of TBI, dose of AED administered, pharmacokinetics and serum levels of AED) may have accounted for the observed disparate prevalence of early PTS.

The studies are even scarcer regarding other AEDs. The effectiveness of valproate vs. short-term phenytoin has been compared for prevention of PTS in patients with ≥ 14 years old. The rates of early PTS were similar when using either valproate or phenytoin (1.5% in the phenytoin treatment group and 4.5% in the valproate arms of the study; p = 0.14). However, a trend showed higher mortality when using valproate. Additionally, the rates of late seizures did not differ among treatment groups.[42] A retrospective analysis of children and adults regarding valproate prophylactic treatment versus no treatment after TBI did not show a significant difference, despite absence of PTS in the treatment group.[43] One single study from 1983 evaluated the use of carbamazepine in severe TBI patients with > 15 years old. It was found that carbamazepine reduced the rate of early PTS by 61% (p < 0.05).[44]

Lastly, it is important to mention a prospective collaborative study on PICU patients admitted after a TBI, involving three American institutions. The study reported that therapies and outcomes vary across different units. However, when applying multivariate models, the authors found that only the use of AED (specific agent not identified) was significantly associated with reduced mortality risk.[45]

Conclusions

The incidence of TBI in children is estimated to be high. PTE has been recognized as one of the most common forms of acquired epilepsies in young people, and it is associated with poor functional and psychosocial outcomes and increased mortality. The pathophysiology of PTE is poorly understood. Different genetic (IL-1β rs1143634 CT genotype and A1AR rs10920573 CT genotype) and neurophysiologic (particularly early sporadic epileptiform discharges) biomarkers seem to be associated with PTE. Potential risk factors that increase the possibility of developing PTE after TBI include or early PTS, higher severity of TBI (i.e., worse GCS, young age, abnormal neuroimaging (subdural hematomas, uncal herniation, brain contusion, skull fractures) and/or prolonged loss of consciousness. Antiepileptic drugs have a role in the prevention of early PTS (up to 7 days) after a severe TBI. However, early treatment with an AED does not protect against the development of PTE. After the diagnosis of PTE has been made, patients benefit from initiating or resuming an antiepileptic drug, in accordance with the usual clinical practice and management. In refractory PTE cases, other interventions such as surgical treatment may be considered.

References

1. Centers for Disease Control and Prevention. Surveillance Report of Traumatic Brain Injury-related Emergency Department Visits, Hospitalizations, and Deaths—United States, 2014. Centers for Disease Control and Prevention, U.S. Department of Health and Human Services. Atlanta, Georgia; 2019.

2. Annegers JF, Grabow JD, Groover RV, et al. Seizures after head trauma: a population study. *Neurology*. 1980;30(7 Pt 1):683–9.

3. Lowenstein DH. Epilepsy after head injury: an overview. *Epilepsia* 2009;50 Suppl 2:4–9.

4. Park JT, Chugani HT. Post-traumatic epilepsy in children-experience from a tertiary referral center. *Pediatr Neurol*. 2015;52(2):174–81.

5. Arndt DH, Lerner JT, Matsumoto JH, et al. Subclinical early posttraumatic seizures detected by continuous EEG monitoring in a consecutive pediatric cohort. *Epilepsia* 2013;54(10):1780–8.

6. Arango JI, Deibert CP, Brown D, Bell M, Dvorchik I, Adelson PD. Posttraumatic seizures in children with severe traumatic brain injury. *Childs Nerv Syst* 2012;28(11):1925–9.

7. Emanuelson I, Uvebrant P. Occurrence of epilepsy during the first 10 years after traumatic brain injury acquired in childhood up to the age of 18 years in the south western Swedish population-based series. *Brain Inj* 2009;23(7):612–6.

8. Hahn YS, Fuchs S, Flannery AM, Barthel MJ, McLone DG. Factors influencing posttraumatic seizures in children. *Neurosurgery* 1988;22(5):864–7.

9. Appleton RE, Demellweek C. Post-traumatic epilepsy in children requiring inpatient rehabilitation following head injury. *J Neurol Neurosurg Psychiatry* 2002;72(5):669–72.

10. Annegers JF, Coan SP. The risks of epilepsy after traumatic brain injury. *Seizure*. 2000;9(7):453–7.

11. Annegers JF, Hauser WA, Coan SP, Rocca WA. A population-based study of seizures after traumatic brain injuries. *N Engl J Med*. 1998;338(1):20–4.

12. Li N, Yang Y, Glover DP, Zhang J, et al. Evidence for impaired plasticity after traumatic brain injury in the developing brain. *J Neurotrauma* 2014;31(4):395–403. www.ncbi.nlm.nih.gov/pubmed/24050267

13. Webster KM, Sun M, Crack P, O'Brien TJ, Shultz SR, Semple BD. Inflammation in epileptogenesis after traumatic brain injury. *J Neuroinflammation* 2017;14(1):10.

14. Ravizza T, Balosso S, Vezzani A. Inflammation and prevention of epileptogenesis. *Neurosci Lett* 2011;497(3):223–30.

15. Peltola J, Palmio J, Korhonen L, et al. Interleukin-6 and interleukin-1 receptor antagonist in cerebrospinal fluid from patients with recent tonic-clonic seizures. *Epilepsy Res* 2000;41(3):205–11.

16. Peltola J, Laaksonen J, Haapala AM, Hurme M, Rainesalo S, Keranen T. Indicators of inflammation after recent tonic-clonic epileptic seizures correlate with plasma interleukin-6 levels. *Seizure* 2002;11(1):44–6.

17. Crespel A, Coubes P, Rousset M-C, et al. Inflammatory reactions in human medial temporal lobe epilepsy with hippocampal sclerosis. *Brain Res* 2002;952(2):159–69.

18. Cotter D, Kelso A, Neligan A. Genetic biomarkers of posttraumatic epilepsy: A systematic review. *Seizure* 2017 Mar;46:53–8.

19. Diamond ML, Ritter AC, Failla MD, et al. IL-1β associations with posttraumatic epilepsy development: a genetics and biomarker cohort study. *Epilepsia* 2014;55(7):1109–19.

20. Wagner AK, Miller MA, Scanlon J, Ren D, Kochanek PM, Conley YP. Adenosine A1 receptor gene variants associated with post-traumatic seizures after severe TBI. *Epilepsy Res* 2010;90(3):259–72.

21. Dadas A, Washington J, Diaz-Arrastia R, Janigro D. Biomarkers in traumatic brain injury (TBI): a review. *Neuropsychiatr Dis Treat* 2018;14:2989–3000.

22. Walker LE, Janigro D, Heinemann U, Riikonen R, Bernard C, Patel M. WONOEP appraisal: Molecular and cellular biomarkers for epilepsy. *Epilepsia* 2016;57(9):1354–62.

23. Angeleri F, Majkowski J, Cacchiò G, et al. Posttraumatic epilepsy risk factors: One-year prospective study after head injury. *Epilepsia* 1999;40:1222–30.

24. Kim JA, Boyle EJ, Wu AC, et al. Epileptiform activity in traumatic brain injury predicts post-traumatic epilepsy. *Ann Neurol* 2018;83(4):858–62.

25. Nordli DR. Varying seizure semiology according to age. *Handb Clin Neurol* 2013;111:455–60.

26. Liesemer K, Bratton SL, Zebrack CM, Brockmeyer D, Statler KD. Early post-traumatic seizures in moderate to severe pediatric traumatic brain injury: rates, risk factors, and clinical features. *J Neurotrauma* 2011;28(5):755–62.

27. Matsumoto JH, Caplan R, McArthur DL, Forgey MJ, Yudovin S, Giza CC. Prevalence of epileptic and nonepileptic events after pediatric traumatic brain injury. *Epilepsy Behav* 2013;27(1):233–7.

28. Keret A, Shweiki M, Bennett-Back O, et al. The clinical characteristics of posttraumatic epilepsy following moderate-to-severe traumatic brain injury in children. *Seizure* 2018;58:29–34.

29. Kochanek PM, Carney N, Adelson PD, et al. Guidelines for the acute medical management of severe traumatic brain injury in infants, children, and adolescents–second edition. *Pediatr Crit Care Med* 2012;13 Suppl 1: S1–82.

30. Kochanek PM, Tasker RC, Carney N, et al. Guidelines for the management of pediatric severe traumatic brain injury, third edition: Update of the Brain Trauma Foundation Guidelines, Executive Summary. *Neurosurgery* 2019;**84**(6):1169–78.

31. Ding K, Gupta PK, Diaz-Arrastia R. Epilepsy after traumatic brain injury. In: Laskowitz D, Grant G, eds. *Translational Research in Traumatic Brain Injury*. Boca Raton (FL), CRC Press; 2016.

32. O'Neill BR, Handler MH, Tong S, Chapman KE. Incidence of seizures on continuous EEG monitoring following traumatic brain injury in children. *J Neurosurg Pediatr* 2015;**16**(2):167–76.

33. Abend NS, Topjian AA, Gutierrez-Colina AM, Donnelly M, Clancy RR, Dlugos DJ. Impact of continuous EEG monitoring on clinical management in critically ill children. *Neurocrit Care* Internet. 2011;**15**(1):70–5. www.ncbi.nlm.nih.gov/pubmed/20499208

34. Herman ST, Abend NS, Bleck TP, et al. Consensus statement on continuous EEG in critically ill adults and children, part I: indications. *J Clin Neurophysiol* 2015;**32**(2):87–95. www.ncbi.nlm.nih.gov/pubmed/25626778

35. Lewis RJ, Yee L, Inkelis SH, Gilmore D. Clinical predictors of post-traumatic seizures in children with head trauma. *Ann Emerg Med* 1993;**22**(7):1114–8.

36. Temkin NR, Dikmen SS, Wilensky AJ, Keihm J, Chabal S, Winn HR. A randomized, double-blind study of phenytoin for the prevention of post-traumatic seizures. *N Engl J Med* 1990;**323**(8):497–502.

37. Inglet S, Baldwin M, Quinones AH, Majercik S, Collingridge DS, MacDonald J. Seizure prophylaxis in patients with traumatic brain injury: A single-center study. *Cureus* 2016; **8**(8):e753–e753.

38. Bhullar IS, Johnson D, Paul JP, Kerwin AJ, Tepas JJ 3rd, Frykberg ER. More harm than good: antiseizure prophylaxis after traumatic brain injury does not decrease seizure rates but may inhibit functional recovery. *J Trauma Acute Care Surg* 2014;**76**(1):51–4.

39. Pearl PL, McCarter R, McGavin CL, et al. Results of phase II levetiracetam trial following acute head injury in children at risk for posttraumatic epilepsy. *Epilepsia* 2013;**54**(9):e135–7.

40. Chung MG, O'Brien NF. Prevalence of early posttraumatic seizures in children with moderate to severe traumatic brain injury despite levetiracetam prophylaxis. *Pediatr Crit Care Med* 2016;**17**(2):150–6.

41. Thapa A, Chandra SP, Sinha S, Sreenivas V, Sharma BS, Tripathi M. Post-traumatic seizures-A prospective study from a tertiary level trauma center in a developing country. *Seizure* 2010;**19**(4):211–6.

42. Temkin NR, Dikmen SS, Anderson GD, et al. Valproate therapy for prevention of posttraumatic seizures: a randomized trial. *J Neurosurg* 1999;**91**(4):593–600.

43. Ma C, Xue Y, Li M, Zhang Y, Li G. Sodium valproate for prevention of early posttraumatic seizures. *Chinese J Traumatol (English edn)* 2010;**13**(5):293–6.

44. Glotzner FL, Haubitz I, Miltner F, Kapp G, Pflughaupt KW. Seizure prevention using carbamazepine following severe brain injuries. *Neurochirurgia (Stuttg)* 1983;**26**(3):66–79[in German].

45. Tilford JM, Simpson PM, Yeh TS, et al. Variation in therapy and outcome for pediatric head trauma patients. *Crit Care Med* 2001;**29**(5):1056–61.

46. Asikainen I, Kaste M, Sarna S. Early and late posttraumatic seizures in traumatic brain injury rehabilitation patients: brain injury factors causing late seizures and influence of seizures on long-term outcome. *Epilepsia* 1999;**40**(5):584–9.

47. Zhao Y, Wu H, Wang X, Li J, Zhang S. Clinical epidemiology of posttraumatic epilepsy in a group of Chinese patients. *Seizure* 2012;**21**(5):322–6.

48. Wang H, Xin T, Sun X, et al. Post-traumatic seizures – a prospective, multicenter, large case study after head injury in China. *Epilepsy Res* 2013;107(3):272–8

Sport-related Concussive Convulsions

Derek D. George, Alan R. Tang, Christopher M. Bonfield
and Aaron M. Yengo-Kahn

Introduction

Sports-related concussion (SRC) has received considerable attention over the last two decades as a significant public health issue. With improved consistency in reporting and efforts geared toward detection and prevention, the incidence of sports-related traumatic brain injuries (TBIs) has recently stabilized in the United States.[1] An understanding of the immediate clinical manifestations of SRC is critical, as early detection, recognition and protocolized action remain the pillars of on-field concussion management. One such immediate clinical manifestation is that of transient abnormal, non-volitional movements. These short-lived, stereotyped movements are known as concussive convulsions. The purpose of this chapter is to discuss the phenomenon of concussive convulsions with special attention paid to sports-related injuries. This chapter will define concussive convulsions and describe the entity's history, pathophysiology and epidemiology. We will also discuss the diagnostic work-up, including electroencephalography (EEG) and neuroimaging. Lastly, practical recommendations for initial management and follow-up will be provided. The decision to focus within the context of sports-related injuries reflects a few important considerations: 1) SRCs are commonly isolated injuries requiring purely clinical diagnosis, therefore, specific attention is directed toward their presentation, and 2) the research surrounding concussive convulsions has relied nearly exclusively on data from sports.

Definition and History

Concussive convulsions were first described by McCrory et al. in 1997 through the observation and review of concussions suffered by Australian rules and rugby league players.[2] Prior to the publication of this study, it had been widely assumed that concussive convulsions were an early manifestation of post-traumatic epilepsy (PTE).[2] However, the authors demonstrated concussive convulsions to be a distinct entity. Retrospectively, eyewitness and video data of 22 concussive convulsions were collected from a 15-year time period. The event descriptions produced from this cohort are now considered the defining features of concussive convulsions. Typically, these convulsions involve a brief tonic phase followed by bilateral myoclonic movements, which were sometimes accompanied by abnormal head movements and/or asymmetric posturing. These episodes were observed to start within two seconds of impact, during a period of loss of consciousness, and lasted a maximum of 150 seconds. Following return of consciousness, athletes were noted to exhibit the typical neurologic and behavioral manifestations of a concussion.[2]

In a subsequent prospective analysis of 102 Australian footballers from McCrory et al. published in 2000, about 25% of concussed athletes showed tonic movements without clonic movements.[3] These initial studies led to an understanding that the semiology of the

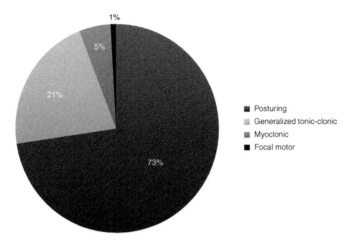

1%
5%
21%
73%

- Posturing
- Generalized tonic-clonic
- Myoclonic
- Focal motor

Figure 6.1 Convulsion semiology
Graphic adapted from Kuhl et al., 2018.[4]

convulsion could vary from athlete to athlete. A 2018 systematic review of 128 cases (7 studies) of sport-related concussive convulsions by Kuhl et al. provided a synopsis of observed semiologies to date. Of these 128 cases, 121 had a recorded semiology (Figure 6.1). Of note, nine of the cases included by Kuhl et al. presented with delayed epilepsy (PTE), and these are not included in Figure 6.1 or in subsequent discussion.

The most common semiology was posturing (88/121; 72.7%), followed by generalized tonic-clonic (26/121; 21.5%), myoclonic (6/121; 5.0%) and focal motor (1/121; 0.8%).[4] Posturing movements described include the "bear-hug" and "righting" reflexes, which most often occur immediately after head impact. Because of the relatively high prevalence of posturing in these cases, recognition of posturing is of utmost importance for quick assessment and stabilization of patients. Although the semiology may change from one concussion to another, the short duration and temporal relationship to a suspected head injury remain the defining features. Thus, we define concussive convulsions as follows:

> Concussive convulsion: an episode of transient, abnormal movement(s), occurring immediately following a head injury and after which an individual returns to a normal or only mildly altered level of consciousness (GCS 13–15). Episodes do not recur in the absence of a repeat head injury.

It should be emphasized that SRC-convulsions are not believed to be a manifestation of post-traumatic epilepsy (PTE). While SRC-convulsions are an isolated, immediate manifestation of head injury, PTE represents one or more unprovoked late post-traumatic seizures occurring after at least one week post-injury.[5] While the incidence of PTE is known to correlate with the severity of injury,[6] a lack of evidence exists for correlation of SRC-convulsions with injury severity.

Pathophysiology

The pathophysiology of SRC convulsions remains largely unknown. The follow-up of study subjects from both investigations by McCrory et al. revealed that players did not have neuroradiologic evidence of TBI or epileptiform discharges on EEG to suggest a structural etiology or epileptogenic foci.[2, 3] McCrory and colleagues therefore concluded that these convulsions were non-epileptic in nature and likely stem from a different pathophysiologic process than PTE.[2] Specifically, McCrory and colleagues drew a similarity between SRC-convulsions and convulsions seen with syncope.

During early investigations of syncopal convulsions, Dell et al. demonstrated that early cerebral hypoxia resulted in direct activation of the reticular activating formation with contemporaneous cortical suppression.[7] This series of hypoxia-related events then results in the tonic and myoclonic movements seen with convulsive syncope.[7, 8] An earlier study by Gastaut and Fischer-Williams had also shown that convulsive syncope did not result in epileptiform EEG changes, as similarly suspected to be the case with concussive convulsions.[9] These elements of convulsive syncope make it appear phenotypically similar to concussive convulsions. However, in the case of concussive convulsions, this transient, functional decerebration is assumed to be initiated immediately by shear forces at the time of impact rather than by a transient period of cortical ischemia (as in syncope), leading to bulbo-pontine reticular formation disinhibition.[8] One hypothesis suggests that strain and shear forces experienced by the ascending reticular activating formation fibers lead to transient functional decerebration.[10] Therefore, while an analogy can be drawn between convulsive syncope and concussive convulsions, the exact pathophysiology remains unknown, and there remains an open investigational opportunity for better pathophysiological understanding.

Epidemiology

Demographic and epidemiologic data on concussive convulsions are lacking due to the relative dearth of studies on the topic. Moreover, published studies have inconsistently recorded important epidemiologic data. As Kuhl et al. reported, basic demographic variables are often incompletely reported. For example, gender was only recorded for 76 of 128 subjects (59.4%) across 7 included studies. Additionally, all of the study subjects were male, making it potentially difficult to generalize findings to other populations.[4] Furthermore, age was recorded for only 27 subjects (21.1%), with an average of 22.9 years. Of note, all these male athletes were engaged in full-contact sports, as defined by the 2008 classification system from the American Academy of Pediatrics.[11]

Regarding the incidence of concussive convulsions, an exact number is not known. In their landmark analysis of eyewitness and video footage from a combined estimated 200,000 player-games across a 15-year period, McCrory et al. identified only 22 cases of concussive convulsion.[2] Their subsequent prospective analysis of 102 concussion cases reported one episode of tonic-clonic movements lasting 150 seconds. However, less lengthy convulsive manifestations were more common: the righting reflex was observed in 40 of 102 subjects (39%), tonic postures in 25 of 102 subjects (25%) and clonic movement in 6 of 102 (6%).[3] In a separate analysis of 35 Youtube™(Google Inc, Mountain View, CA;) videos showing concussive events, Hosseini et al. reported 23 instances (66%) of tonic posturing known as the fencing response. There were no noted tonic-clonic convulsive events.[12] Based on these studies, it can be concluded that concussive convulsion manifestations, including posturing, clonic movements and the righting reflex occur commonly in the immediate post-injury period, while tonic-clonic convulsions are a rarer consequence of head injury.

Diagnosis and Further Work-Up

As discussed above, the diagnosis of concussive convulsions is largely clinical and relies upon a careful history and description of the observed convulsion semiology. Adjuncts such as EEG and neuroimaging have been evaluated in individuals who suffered concussive convulsions and the negative findings do require a brief mention to fully understand the practical nature of the work-up.

Electroencephalogram

Through systematic review, Kuhl et al. report that EEG was performed in 23 (19%) of 121 cases.[4] Although no EEG data were obtained during the actual convulsive events, EEGs performed in the post-convulsion period did not show abnormalities in 22/23 athletes who had concussive convulsions.[4] One Australian rules footballer demonstrated transient slowing (without any suggestion of epileptogenicity) in the left temporal lobe immediately after injury, but follow-up EEGs at one week and 24 months post-injury revealed no epileptiform discharges or slowing.[2] Based on these findings, the role of EEG in the work-up of concussive convulsions is limited. Athletes who suffer a concussive convulsion are highly unlikely to demonstrate EEG abnormalities consistent with epileptogenic foci. That said, EEG may be considered if the convulsive event is not immediately following the injury, that is, convulsions occur in a delayed manner. EEG should also be considered if an unprovoked convulsion occurs separate from the traumatic event. In both situations, the concern is the presence of another etiology for the seizures, as delayed seizures are unlikely to be related to a single concussion.

Neuroimaging

Neuroimaging has been performed in 31 of 121 (25.6%) reported cases of concussive convulsions, with the most common modality being head computerized tomography (CT) in 15 of 31 (48.3%) cases.[4] Head magnetic resonance imaging (MRI) was performed in 14 of 31 (45.2%) cases. Cervical radiographs were captured in 2 cases (6.5%). Neuroimaging did not demonstrate any identifiable intracranial pathology in any of the 121 cases of concussive convulsion reported in the literature, suggesting that imaging is of limited utility in the workup of isolated concussive convulsions.[4] Conversely, imaging studies should be considered if a seizure develops in a delayed fashion relative to the injury or if repeated unprovoked convulsions occur, as these symptoms may indicate an alternative etiology of seizures. Additionally, neuroimaging should be pursued in anyone with a Glasgow Coma Score (GCS) less than 13, a focal neurologic deficit or other signs and symptoms concerning for increased intracranial pressure such as persistent projectile vomiting, progressive severe headache and/or somnolence. The data on the work-up and management of reported cases of concussive convulsions are summarized in Table 6.1.

Management

Anti-epileptic Drugs

Despite limited data, it appears clear that anti-epileptic drugs (AED) are not required after sports-related concussive convulsion. There have been no epileptogenic abnormalities reported on EEG, supporting the notion that AEDs are unnecessary. However, it is key to understand the limitations of EEG monitoring and imaging studies. Thus far, no

Table 6.1 Semiology, diagnosis and management of 121 cases of concussive convulsions

Clinical presentation	Number of participants (%)
Seizure semiology	
Posturing	88 (72.7)
Generalized tonic-clonic	26 (21.5)
Myoclonic	6 (5)
Focal motor	1 (0.8)
Diagnosis	
Electroencephalogram	
Performed	23 (19)
Normal intracranial findings	23 (19)
bnormal intracranial findings	0 (0)
Not performed	98 (81)
Imaging studies	
No imaging or not reported	90 (74.4)
Head computed tomography	15 (12.4)
Positive findings	0
Head magnetic resonance imaging	14 (11.6)
Positive findings	0
Cervical plain radiograph	2 (1.7)
Positive findings	0
Management	
Antiepileptic drugs	
Prescribed	1 (0.8)
Not prescribed or not reported	120 (99.2)
Follow-up	
Outpatient setting[a]	
Average follow-up time	3.2 years
Return-to-play[b]	
Average time to return-of-play	14.8 days

[a] Follow-up was only reported in 18 of 121 cases
[b] Return-to-play was only reported in 25 of 121 cases
These data were adapted from Kuhl et al., 2018[4]

studies have reported EEGs obtained during the concussive convulsion episode. Furthermore, there are very few studies that document longitudinal follow-up after a concussive convulsion. Even with these limitations, our recommendation remains to withhold AED administration for a typical concussive convulsion. In cases that do not follow the typical presentation of a concussive convulsion, such as delayed seizures, we would recommend treating in alignment with standard management of a first-time seizure.

For example, Meehan et al. reported a case involving the management of a head injury acquired during a wrestling match using AEDs.[13] The patient presented to the emergency department 40 minutes after the incident with continued focal myoclonus of the right forearm and hand, in addition to altered mental status. One milligram of lorazepam and one gram of fosphenytoin were prescribed; the seizure activity subsided after the patient received these medications, and all imaging, including head CT and basic laboratory studies performed were negative. No long-term AEDs were prescribed to the patient, and an MRI of the brain 2 weeks later was also negative. The length of this presentation contrasts significantly from the typical transient concussive convulsion that lasts well under 5 minutes and thus requires individualized treatment considerations such as neuroimaging and AED administration.

Follow-up Neuroimaging and EEG

As discussed above, there are no reported epileptogenic EEG findings or neuroimaging findings after a standard concussive convulsion. In light of this, there is no need for scheduling of outpatient follow-up EEG or neuroimaging unless a new separate clinical concern arises. If a new seizure occurs or any focal deficit or altered mental status occurs in a delayed manner after the suspected head injury, we would recommend urgent evaluation with standard neuroimaging, such as a CT scan of the head. An EEG may be obtained if dictated by history and physical yet would not be required simply given the history of concussive convulsion.

General Clinic Follow-up

It is essential for patients presenting with concussive convulsions to comply with regimented and regular follow-up schedules as with any concussed patient. Those that participate in organized sports may require (depending on their home state or country legislation) clearance by a medical doctor (MD or doctor of osteopathic medicine), which requires an in-person visit. Generally, routine follow-up for the concussion should be the same regardless of the presence of concussive convulsion. There is no evidence to schedule more frequent or a longer course of visits in general if the patient suffered a concussive convulsion.

Conclusion

Sport-related concussive convulsions are uncommonly seen after a concussion. For a patient presenting with a concussive convulsion, there is no evidence of positive imaging studies, abnormal EEGs, long-term sequelae or a need for AED prescriptions. However, one must adhere to the strict definition of concussive convulsions – transient convulsive or tonic events occurring immediately after a head impact and should certainly cease in well under 5 minutes with the athlete returning to reasonable mental status (GCS 13–15). If the event is delayed after the head impact or unprovoked, further work-up with neuroimaging and potentially EEG is necessary. Presently, standard sport-related concussive convulsions do not require any additional care outside of typical sport-related concussion management.

References

1. Sarmiento K, Thomas KE, Daugherty J, et al. Emergency department visits for sports-and recreation-related traumatic brain injuries among children—United States, 2010–2016. *Morbidity and Mortality Weekly Report* 2019;**68**(10):237.

2. McCrory PR, Bladin PF, Berkovic SF. Retrospective study of concussive convulsions in elite Australian rules and rugby league footballers: phenomenology, aetiology, and outcome. *BMJ* 1997;**314**(7075):171.

3. McCrory PR, Berkovic SF. Video analysis of acute motor and convulsive manifestations in sport-related concussion. *Neurology.* 2000;**54**(7):1488–91.

4. Kuhl NO, Yengo-Kahn AM, Burnette H, Solomon GS, Zuckerman SL. Sport-related concussive convulsions: a systematic review. *Phys Sportsmed* 2018;**46**(1):1–7.

5. Jennett B. Early traumatic epilepsy: incidence and significance after nonmissile injuries. *Arch Neurol* 1974;**30**(5):394–8.

6. Verellen RM, Cavazos JE. Post-traumatic epilepsy: an overview. *Therapy* 2010;**7**(5):527–31.

7. Dell P, Hugelin A, Bonvallet M. Effects of hypoxia on the reticular and cortical diffuse systems. In: *Cerebral Anoxia and the Electroencephalogram* (ed Gastaut H, Meyer JS): 46–58. Springfield: Charles C Thomas, 1961.

8. McCrory PR, Berkovic SF. Concussive convulsions. *Sports Med* 1998;**25**(2):131–6.

9. Gastaut H, Fischer-Williams M. Electro-encephalographic study of syncope; its differentiation from epilepsy. *Lancet* 1957;**273**(7004):1018–25.

10. Steenerson K, Starling AJ. Pathophysiology of sports-related concussion. *Neurologic Clinics.* 2017;**35**(3):403–8.

11. Rice SG. Medical conditions affecting sports participation. *Pediatrics* 2008;**121**(4):841–8.

12. Hosseini AH, Lifshitz J. Brain injury forces of moderate magnitude elicit the fencing response. *Med Sci Sports Exerc.* 2009;**41**(9):1687–97.

13. Meehan WP, Hoppa E, Capraro AJ. Case report: Focal motor seizure in a wrestler with a sport-related concussion. *Phys Sportsmed* 2008;**36**(1):125–8.

Chapter 7

Accidents and Injuries during Seizures

Simona Lattanzi and Vincenzo Belcastro

Introduction

Research and clinical experience suggest that people with epilepsy are more likely than the general population to have accidents and related injuries, including bone fractures, wounds and lacerations, abrasions, head trauma, concussion, drowning, burns, sprains/strains, broken teeth and eye lesions.[1, 7]

The home, street and workplace are, in decreasing order, the leading sites where accidents and injuries occur.[1] Most accidents and injuries are fairly mild to moderate in severity and uncomplicated. In rare circumstances, these events can be fatal, mostly motor vehicle accidents, drownings, severe falls and burns.[1] Even injuries that do not prove lethal can be the cause of disability, missed work or school, health care expenses and indirect costs.

Some of the accidents and injuries can be directly attributed to seizures (Figure 7.1). Indeed, seizures can be associated with alterations or impairment of consciousness and loss of motor control. Additional injuries may be the consequence of seizures themselves, as for example shoulder dislocation due to muscle contraction during a generalized tonic-clonic seizure or tongue biting from contraction of masseter muscles.[8, 9]

Comorbid conditions and concurrent handicaps, neurological and cognitive deficits, behavioural and psychiatric disorders as well as side effects of antiepileptic medications, like drowsiness, ataxia, blurred vision and diplopia, may be present in patients with epilepsy and act as independent putative causes of accidents and injuries; impaired judgement or

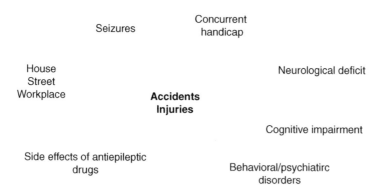

Figure 7.1 Risk factors for accidents and injuries in patients with epilepsy.

vigilance, impulsiveness, sleepiness and poor balance are potential underlying mechanisms (Figure 7.1).[1, 10–12]

Motor Vehicle Accidents in Patients with Epilepsy

There is considerable variation across individual studies in the rates of motor vehicle accidents reported in patients with epilepsy. In a recently published systematic review that included 30 observational studies, the prevalence of traffic accidents ranged from 0 to 61%.[13] Remarkably, studies recruited patients with a wide range of seizure disorders and baseline characteristics, including first seizure, childhood onset epilepsy, drug-resistant epilepsy, people collected by a free ambulance service, patients on at least one antiepileptic agent or dependent on psychoactive drugs.[13] One third of the studies specified the time frame considered to estimate prevalence, which covered the past 1, 2, 3, 4, 5 or 10 years.[13] Only half of the study authors described whether the traffic accidents were seizure-related or not, and the proportion of accidents due to an actual seizure versus a driver error remained difficult to ascertain in many cases.[13] Studies were predominantly performed in high-income settings, limiting the generalizability of the evidence to middle and low-income countries, which are characterized by higher incidence of epilepsy and road traffic fatality rate.[14, 15] Furthermore, in high-income countries about 90% of patients with epilepsy drive before and near all hold a driver's licence ten years after the disease onset, whereas only 20–30% of people with epilepsy drive in middle-income countries.[16–18]

The existing literature suggests that people with epilepsy are overall more likely to be involved in motor vehicle accidents than the unaffected population with a risk that ranges from 1.2 to 2.1 in different study populations.[1, 11, 19–23] By contrast, no difference in risk of accidents was found between epileptic and non-epileptic drivers in a retrospective questionnaire survey in the UK.[24] Potential underestimation bias could explain such discrepancy as drivers in the UK are required to self-report to the authorities any medical condition that can affect driving ability.

It is worth noting that people with epilepsy also have a 2.2- and 1.7-fold increased risk of pedestrian and bicycle accidents, respectively in comparison to controls.[19]

Some studies tried to elaborate on the nature of motor vehicle accidents in people with epilepsy. In this regard, accidents related to epilepsy have been reported to produce more minor injuries, and to be more likely to involve a single vehicle, carry a sole occupant, begin mostly with an 'out of control movement', to be a collision with a fixed object, involve an 'off path, on straight' mechanism and occur in less densely populated areas than non-seizure related crashes.[25, 26] Moreover, crashes related to generalized epilepsy have been shown to involve younger drivers and seizure-provoking factors and occur earlier during the day in comparison to focal epilepsy.[26]

Protective factors against motor vehicle accidents include a prolonged seizure-free interval, epilepsy surgery, presence of reliable auras, history of few non-seizure related crashes and regular adjustment of antiepileptic therapy.[27, 28] Patients with a seizure-free interval of 6 months have a 85% reduced risk of accident compared to subjects with shorter intervals, and the risk is reduced by more than 90% in patients with >12 months of freedom from seizures.[28] Conversely, non-adherence and poor compliance to the antiepileptic drug regimen and driving in violation of restrictions are associated with a higher risk of traffic crashes.[26, 29–31]

The use of newer versus older antiepileptic drugs, namely lamotrigine or levetiracetam versus carbamazepine or oxcarbazepine, did not affect the risk of serious motor vehicle accidents in a Swedish nationwide cohort study. This suggests how adherence to antiepileptic therapy may be emphasized over the choice of a specific agent in counselling patients about driving to minimize the risk of seizures and car crashes.[19] A nested case–control study performed in the Australian state of Victoria also identified that, although 20% of patients with epilepsy had a car accident before the diagnosis, approximately one fifth of seizure-induced crashes were attributable to non-compliance to antiepileptic treatment once prescribed.[26] A retrospective open-cohort study using Medicaid claims data from Florida, Iowa and New Jersey found that non-adherence to therapy was associated with a significantly higher incidence of motor vehicle injuries than adherence in adult patients who had a diagnosis of epilepsy and had been prescribed antiepileptic drugs.[32]

Driving restriction is a major critical issue in patients with epilepsy. Worldwide, in order to balance the economic and social relevance of having a driving licence with the hazard to public safety, the main assumption that inspires current legislation is to reduce rather than avoid risks by allowing people with an acceptable low likelihood of a seizure-related traffic accident to drive.[2] Seizure-free interval is the main measure and dominating factor to establish fitness to drive and the time since the last seizure represents the major or sole criterion employed most widely by driver-licencing authorities.[33] A great variability, however, exists in the specific rules and driving restrictions across countries and even within states in the USA and European Union. Additional variables that can predict the risk of seizure recurrence and seizure-related accidents include age, seizure type, diurnal pattern, seizure duration and electroencephalographic abnormalities.[34–36]

Treatment withdrawal may be indicated in people with epilepsy in remission. In this regard, the Medical Research Council antiepileptic drug withdrawal study, which involved 1,021 patients with epilepsy, found a risk of 30% for seizure recurrence in the next 12 months immediately following drug taper.[37] Further, the risk of seizure after drug tapering decreases with the increasing of the seizure-free interval.[37–39] In the case of seizure recurrence, when treatment was reinstated, the risk of a seizure in the following 12 months was 26%, 18% and 17% after 3, 6 and 12 months spent without seizures.[37] These figures should be born in mind when advising time off driving after discontinuation of antiepileptic drugs. In the UK, people with epilepsy are advised to not drive during drug tapering and for the next 6 months[40]; in the USA, no laws exist about driving restriction during or after drug tapering, but 80% of epilepsy specialists would advise to not drive for 3 months after treatment withdrawal.[41]

There is converging evidence that people with epilepsy who are compliant with local driving restrictions have a risk of traffic accidents that is similar to that observed in the general population, and most epilepsy patients causing motor vehicle crashes did not fulfil the criteria established by law.[42–44] It is, hence, of great concern to know that only around half of patients with epilepsy are aware of the rules regarding driving privileges,[45, 46] and up to two-fifths of people with seizures drive without meeting the seizure freedom requirement.[47, 48]

Seizure-related Injuries

Seizure-related injuries have been classified into burns, head trauma, dental traumas, fractures, major body injuries, penetrating traumas, road injuries and drowning.[12, 49, 50]

Noteworthy, a patient could have one or more injuries at different body locations during a seizure or multiple injuries with different seizures.

A number of studies have shown that head traumas are the most frequent types of injury, followed by fractures.[50–54] In a recent study by Lagunju et al., 57 children (46%) had a seizure-related injury and 31 (25%) of them presented multiple injuries; higher seizure frequency was reported as the main risk factor for seizure-related injuries.[52]

Head injuries usually result from falls occurring during seizures. The patient can fully recover from trauma, but cognitive and psychological symptoms may persist over time. The risk of fractures has been also shown to be increased in patients with epilepsy. The risk of fractures of the extremities due to seizures has been reported to be 2.4 times higher in patients with epilepsy, and bone fractures showed a rate of 19%.[9, 55] In addition, patients with epilepsy can further become more prone to have fractures due to the osteopenic effects of some antiepileptic medications, mainly those of the first generation.[55]

A recent study showed that patients with epilepsy tend to have multiple injuries and most of these injuries occur during everyday activities at home.[54] The most common type of seizure-related injury that happens at home is dental trauma, followed by burns and head traumas. The most common injuries occurring outdoor result in fractures, followed by head and body traumas, including lacerations and soft tissue injuries.[54] In a multicentre prospective study, the probability of seizure-related injuries was significantly greater in the domestic environment than on the street or at work.[56] These results may be, at least partly, attributed to the decreased level of alertness and attention to safety in domestic places as well as to the tendency of epileptic patients to spend more time at home and isolate themselves due to the fear of presenting seizures in public. The evidence that home is the main setting of possible serious injuries also highlights the need to take adequate preventive measures to minimize risks.

Conclusion

Quality of life is defined as the individual's perception of physical health, psychological state and level of independence, social relationships and personal beliefs. Accidents and injuries that occur during seizures may require hospitalization, cause disability, influence the ability to drive and restrict holding a driving licence, increase loss of work productivity, increase indirect costs, decrease self-esteem, contribute to social stigmatization and, hence, affect the overall quality of life in patients with epilepsy.[9]

The knowledge of the nature and risk factors for accidents and injuries that most commonly occur in people with epilepsy represents the key step to adequately counsel and inform both patients and their families or caregivers and adopt reliable preventive measures. Most accidents and injuries occur within the first 2 years of the diagnosis of epilepsy, which is the period associated with the most significant adjustment in management and the greatest risk of seizure recurrence.[10, 11] Lower educational level has been demonstrated to be a meaningful risk factor of having seizure-related injuries.[54] The remarkable prevalence of seizure-related injuries among patients with poor education is a further signal that epilepsy-related risks are still overlooked and their underappreciation can have major socioeconomic impact. Awareness-raising campaigns and education need to be boosted among both health care professionals and lay population to promote and increase the knowledge on epilepsy-related issues.

References

1. Beghi E. Accidents and injuries in patients with epilepsy. *Expert Rev Neurother* 2009;9:291–8.

2. Tomson T, Beghi E, Sundqvist A, Johannessen SI. Medical risks in epilepsy: a review with focus on physical injuries, mortality, traffic accidents and their prevention. *Epilepsy Res* 2004;60:1–16.

3. Kwon CS, Liu M, Quan H, et al. The incidence of injuries in persons with and without epilepsy–a population-based study. *Epilepsia* 2010;51:2247–53.

4. Neufeld MY, Vishne T, Chistik V, Korczyn AD. Life-long history of injuries related to seizures. *Epilepsy Res* 1999;34:123–7.

5. Buck D, Baker GA, Jacoby A, Smith DF, Chadwick DW. Patients' experiences of injury as a result of epilepsy. *Epilepsia* 1997;38:439–44.

6. Kirby S, Sadler RM. Injury and death as a result of seizures. *Epilepsia* 1995;36:25–8.

7. van den Broek M, Beghi E, RESt-1 Group. Accidents in patients with epilepsy: types, circumstances, and complications: a European cohort study. *Epilepsia* 2004;45:667–72.

8. Gosens T, Poels PJE, Rondhuis JJ. Posterior dislocation fractures of the shoulder in seizure disorders—two case reports and a review of literature. *Seizure* 2000;9:446–8.

9. Camfield C, Camfield P. Injuries from seizures are a serious, persistent problem in childhood onset epilepsy: a population-based study. *Seizure* 2015;27:80–3.

10. Krumholz A, Wiebe S, Gronseth GS, et al. Evidence-based guideline: Management of an unprovoked first seizure in adults: Report of the Guideline Development Subcommittee of the American Academy of Neurology and the American Epilepsy Society. *Neurology* 2015;84:1705–13.

11. Mahler B, Carlsson S, Andersson T, Tomson T. Risk for injuries and accidents in epilepsy: A prospective population-based cohort study. *Neurology.* 2018;90:e779–89.

12. Asadi-Pooya AA, Nikseresht A, Yaghoubi E, Nei M. Physical injuries in patients with epilepsy and their associated risk factors. *Seizure* 2012;21:165–8.

13. Xu Y, Shanthosh J, Zhou Z, et al. Prevalence of driving and traffic accidents among people with seizures: A systematic review. *Neuroepidemiology* 2019;53:1–12.

14. Kotsopoulos IA, van Merode T, Kessels FG, de Krom MC, Knottnerus JA. Systematic review and meta-analysis of incidence studies of epilepsy and unprovoked seizures. *Epilepsia* 2002;43:1402–9.

15. World Health Organization. Global status report on road safety 2013: supporting a decade of action. Available from: www.who.int/violence_injury_prevention/road_safety_status/2013/report/en/. Accessed December 2019.

16. Perucca P, Hesdorffer DC, Gilliam FG. Response to first antiepileptic drug trial predicts health outcome in epilepsy. *Epilepsia* 2011; 52: 2209–15.

17. Lindsten H, Stenlund H, Forsgren L. Leisure time and social activity after a newly diagnosed unprovoked epileptic seizure in adult age. A population-based case referent study. *Acta Neurol Scand* 2003;107:125–33.

18. Chen J, Yan B, Lu H, et al. Driving among patients with epilepsy in West China. *Epilepsy Behav* 2014;33:1–6.

19. Sundelin HEK, Chang Z, Larsson H, et al. Epilepsy, antiepileptic drugs, and serious transport accidents: a nationwide cohort study. *Neurology* 2018;90:e1111–8.

20. Hormia A. Does epilepsy mean higher susceptibility to traffic accidents. *Acta Psychiatr Scand Suppl* 1961;36:210–2.

21. Keys JG, Martin CJ Jr, Barrow RL, Fabing HD. The epileptic automobile driver in Ohio. *Ohio State Med J* 1961;57:1127–31.

22. Waller JA. Chronic medical conditions and traffic safety: review of the California experience. *N Engl J Med* 1965;273:413–20.

23. Hansotia P, Broste SK. The effect of epilepsy or diabetes mellitus on the risk of

automobile accidents. *N Engl J Med* 1991;**324**:22–6.

24. Taylor J, Chadwick D, Johnson T. Risk of accidents in drivers with epilepsy. *J Neurol Neurosurg Psychiatry* 1996;**60**:621–7.

25. Andermann F, Rémillard GM, Zifkin BG, Trottier AG, Drouin P. Epilepsy and driving. *Can J Neurol Sci* 1988;**15**:371–7.

26. Neal A, Carne R, Odell M, Ballek D, D'Souza WJ, Cook MJ. Characteristics of motor vehicle crashes associated with seizure: car crash semiology. *Neurology* 2018;**91**: e1102–11.

27. Classen S, Crizzle AM, Winter SM, Silver W, Eisenschenk S. Evidence-based review on epilepsy and driving. *Epilepsy Behav* 2012; **23**: 103–12.

28. Krauss GL, Krumholz A, Carter RC, Li G, Kaplan P. Risk factors for seizure-related motor vehicle crashes in patients with epilepsy. *Neurology* 1999;**52**:1324–9.

29. Sheth SG, Krauss G, Krumholz A, Li G. Mortality in epilepsy: driving fatalities vs other causes of death in patients with epilepsy. *Neurology* 2004;**63**:1002–7.

30. Berg AT, Vickrey BG, Sperling MR, et al. Driving in adults with refractory localization-related epilepsy. Multi-Center Study of Epilepsy Surgery. *Neurology* 2000;**54**:625–30.

31. Sillanpää M, Shinnar S. Obtaining a driver's license and seizure relapse in patients with childhood-onset epilepsy. *Neurology* 2005;**64**:680–6.

32. Faught E, Duh MS, Weiner JR, Guerin A, Cunnington MC. Nonadherence to antiepileptic drugs and increased mortality: findings from the RANSOM Study. *Neurology* 2008;**71**:1572–78.

33. Fisher RS, Drazkowski JF. A comment on driving and neurologic impairment. *Mayo Clin Proc* 2017; **92**: 1326–7.

34. Gastaut H, Zifkin BG. The risk of automobile accidents with seizures occurring while driving: relation to seizure type. *Neurology* 1987; **37**: 1613–6.

35. Bonnett LJ, Tudur-Smith C, Williamson PR, Marson AG. Risk of recurrence after a first seizure and implications for driving: further analysis of the multicentre study of early epilepsy and single seizures. *BMJ* 2010;**341**:c6477.

36. Fisher RS, Parsonage M, Beaussart M et al. Epilepsy and driving: an international perspective. *Epilepsia* 1994;**35**:675–84.

37. Bonnett LJ, Shukralla A, Tudur-Smith C, Williamson PR, Marson AG. Seizure recurrence after antiepileptic drug withdrawal and the implications for driving: further results from the MRC Antiepileptic Drug Withdrawal Study and a systematic review. *J Neurol Neurosurg Psychr* 2011;**82**:1328–33.

38. Lossius MI, Hessen E, Mowinckel P, et al. Consequences of antiepileptic drug withdrawal: a randomized, double-blind study (Akershus Study). *Epilepsia* 2008;**49**: 455–63.

39. Specchio LM, Beghi E. Should antiepileptic drugs be withdrawn in seizure-free patients? *CNS Drugs* 2004;**18**:201–12.

40. Gislason T, Tomasson K, Reynisdottir H, Bjornsson JK, Kristbjarnarson H. Medical risk factors amongst drivers in single-car accidents. *J Intern Med* 1997;**241**:213–9.

41. Joshi CN, Vossler DG, Spanaki M, Draszowki JF, Towne AR; Members of the Treatments Committee of the American Epilepsy Society. "Chance takers are accident makers": Are patients with epilepsy really taking a chance when they drive? *Epilepsy Curr* 2019;**19**:221–6.

42. Mintzer S. Driven to tears: epilepsy specialists and the automobile. *Epilepsy Curr* 2015;**15**:279–82.

43. Hansotia P. Automobile driving and epilepsy: a medical perspective. *Wis Med J* 1991;**90**:112–5.

44. Thorbecke R. Epilepsy and driving license in the Federal Republic of Germany and other European countries. *Jpn J Psychiatry Neurol* 1991;**45**:313–7.

45. Elliott JO, Long L. Perceived risk, resources, and perceptions concerning driving and epilepsy: a patient perspective. *Epilepsy Behav* 2008;**13**:381–6.

46. Zis P, Siatouni A, Kimiskidis VK, et al. Disobedience and driving in patients with

epilepsy in Greece. *Epilepsy Behav* 2014;**41**:179–82.

47. Hasegawa S, Kumagai K, Kaji S. Epilepsy and driving: a survey of automobile accidents attributed to seizure. *Jpn J Psychiatry Neurol* 1991;**45**:327–31.

48. Takeda A, Kawai I, Fukushima Y, Yagi K. Driving and epilepsy: a prospective questionnaire survey in Japan. Committee on Driver's Licenses, the Japan Epilepsy Society, Shizuoka. *Jpn J Psychiatry Neurol* 1991;**45**:319–22.

49. Friedman DE, Tobias RS, Akman CI, Smith EO, Levin HS. Recurrent seizure-related injuries in people with epilepsy at a tertiary epilepsy center: a 2-year longitudinal study. *EpilepsyBehav* 2010;**19**:400–4.

50. Prasad V, Kendrick D, Sayal K, Thomas SL, West J. Injury among children and young adults with epilepsy. *Pediatrics* 2014;**133**: 827–35.

51. Buck D, Baker GA, Jacoby A, Smith DF, Chadwick DW. Patients' experiences of injury as a result of epilepsy. *Epilepsia* 1997;**38**:439–44.

52. Lagunju IA, Oyinlade AO, Babatunde OD. Seizure-related injuries in children and adolescents with epilepsy. *EpilepsyBehav* 2016;**54**:131–4.

53. Neufeld MY, Vishne T, Chistik V, Korczyn AD. Life-long history of injuries related to seizures. *Epilepsy Res* 1999;**34**:123–7.

54. Cengiz O, Atalar AÇ, Tekin B, Bebek N, Baykan B, Gürses C. Impact of seizure-related injuries on quality of life. *Neurol Sci* 2019;**40**:577–83.

55. Persson HB, Alberts KA, Farahmand BY, Tomson T. Risk of extremity fractures in adult outpatients with epilepsy. *Epilepsia* 2002;**43**:768–72.

56. van den Broek M, Beghi E. Accidents in patients with epilepsy: types, circumstances, and complications: a European cohort study. *Epilepsia* 2004;**45**:667–72.

Chapter

8

Cognitive Rehabilitation of Traumatic Brain Injury and Post-traumatic Epilepsy

Sarah E. Hall, Genevieve Rayner and Sarah J. Wilson

Introduction

In a small number of people, the shock and disability that stems from having incurred a traumatic brain injury (TBI) is compounded by the emergence of post-traumatic epilepsy (PTE). As detailed in earlier chapters of this book, PTE is defined as one or more unprovoked seizures that manifest at least a week after TBI.[1] Risk factors encompass TBI-related features such as injury severity, intracerebral haemorrhage, penetrating injuries and early post-traumatic seizures, as well as factors related to the individual such as older age at the time of injury, a family history of epilepsy, genetic features like the ApoE-ε4 allele of apolipoprotein E and premorbid psychiatric illness.[2, 3]

There is growing speculation that the emergence of PTE after a head injury represents a 'double hit' to cognitive functioning, whereby the neurocognitive substrates or networks damaged by the primary trauma are further undermined by a disease characterised by acute-on-chronic disturbance to these same systems (see Semple *et al.*, 2019[4] for a recent review). There remains, however, a limited number of sources empirically delineating the cognitive and behavioural sequelae of PTE specifically. As such this chapter integrates findings from the parallel neuropsychology literatures investigating TBI and epilepsy to supplement our review of the extant PTE research.

Presented here is a model of cognitive decrement in adults with PTE that is framed in terms of diffuse disruption to neurocognitive brain networks caused by the primary TBI and in some cases then additionally undermined by the development of epilepsy. In light of the scarcity of empirical studies, it is reasonable to assume that the secondary mechanism for neurocognitive decrement attributable to the epilepsy is multifactorial. As in primary epilepsy, cognitive impairment in PTE could stem from seizures and interictal epileptic discharges kindling and propagating along the same neurocognitive networks damaged by the TBI,[5, 6] changes to the topography or connectivity of networks hijacked by seizures,[7, 8] or perhaps even a shared genetic mechanism underlying vulnerability to PTE and neurocognitive deficits. There may also be significant secondary psychosocial consequences of PTE exacerbated by behavioural difficulties accompanying TBI, such as disruption to educational, vocational and social development, further impacting cognition.

This chapter also outlines an approach to cognitive remediation for people with PTE adapted from the well-established principles of neuropsychological rehabilitation for TBI and supplemented by the more circumscribed epilepsy rehabilitation literature. In recognition of the multidetermined nature of cognitive deficits in PTE, this rehabilitation approach takes into account the relative contributions of structural brain damage, functional network dysfunction and neurological and psychiatric symptomatology, as well as the psychological and social adjustment processes that commonly accompany this condition.

Primary Cognitive Consequences of TBI

As introduced in earlier chapters, TBI occurs due to blunt head trauma in which the head is struck or moved violently. This physical force triggers a range of complex pathophysiological mechanisms that exert differential effects on neurological injury and repair. Primary effects occur at the time of the acute injury when tissues and blood vessels are damaged, compressed, stretched or torn, and they also include processes of neuronal cell death and Wallerian degeneration.[9] These primary effects trigger a complex cascade of secondary pathophysiological effects that evolve over time and space, further altering neuronal activity and connections.[10] The resulting damage can be both focal and diffuse in nature, impacting key brain structures as well as widespread networks that underpin a range of cognitive functions.

Prefrontal structures, especially those on the orbital surfaces, are particularly vulnerable to focal damage due to their proximity to bony protuberances inside the skull.[11, 12] The orbitofrontal region plays a key role in inhibitory control, social awareness and judgement and understanding of the consequences of behaviour.[13, 14] Consequently, many individuals with TBI have difficulty anticipating the consequences of their actions and monitoring and adjusting behaviour in line with goals and social expectations in complex 'real-world' situations.[15–19] This can be compounded by deficits in 'cold' executive functions, including planning, problem-solving, idea generation, cognitive flexibility and abstract thinking, that can emerge following damage to dorsolateral prefrontal cortex and associated networks.[20, 21]

Diffuse axonal injury (DAI) occurs when there is stretching and shearing of axons due to acceleration–deceleration forces, leading to widespread damage to white matter tracts.[22] The extent of the damage depends on the nature and severity of the injury, with more pronounced white matter volume loss resulting from more severe injuries.[23] Cognitively, DAI can disconnect broadly distributed networks that underpin complex functions including attention, memory and executive function, as well as undermine speed of information processing, contributing to poorer functional outcomes.[24, 25] As such, the typical cognitive picture after severe TBI with DAI is of slow and effortful information processing that is vulnerable to distraction and highly susceptible to fatigue.[26]

In addition to cognitive deficits in attention, memory, speed of information processing and executive functioning, TBI can also lead to problems recognising emotions,[27–31] identifying and labelling one's own emotions,[32–34] and understanding others' emotions, affective states and feelings (i.e. affective theory of mind or cognitive empathy).[35–37] This likely reflects damage to a broadly distributed fronto-temporo-parietal network involved in social cognition, which is vulnerable to disruption after TBI.[11, 12, 38–40] These difficulties can have a profound impact on a person's daily life, leading to misinterpretation of the behaviours and actions of others[34, 42, 43] and socially inappropriate behaviours,[44] particularly when executive problems such as disinhibition and impulsivity are also present.[45] Impaired self-awareness further complicates this picture, with many individuals unable to recognise changes in their emotions and behaviour,[46] ultimately contributing to growing social disconnection and loneliness.

For instance, these difficulties can negatively impact an individual's ability to maintain close relationships and interact appropriately with carers, family, friends and colleagues.[47] A previously caring father and husband might be described as aloof and dismissive post injury; some partners liken it to having another child in the family.[48] Individuals with TBI may start to withdraw from others because socialising is stressful and tiring, with family reporting that they are spending most of the day alone in their room or watching television for hours on end.[26] Others may find this behaviour difficult to understand, contributing to further relationship breakdown.[49] Friends may gradually make less of an effort to maintain friendships, and social networks can shrink over time, leading to social isolation.[50] The case vignette of 'Shane' illustrates some of the social and occupational challenges that can arise after severe TBI.

Case Vignette 1: 'Shane' Executive dysfunction and social problems after severe TBI

Medical and psychosocial history. Shane is a 61-year-old man who was working full-time as the director of a successful mechanic business prior to his injury. He is married with two adult children. His medical history includes hypertension and moderate alcohol use.

Injury details. Shane sustained a severe TBI following an alleged assault in a bar, in which his head struck the concrete pavement. Glasgow Coma Scale score at the scene was 7. Shane's acute injuries included a right subdural haemorrhage with 2 mm midline shift, a small right frontal and temporal sub-arachnoid haemorrhage, fractured right petrous temporal bone and multiple cerebral contusions. He spent 16 days in the acute hospital, including 13 days in ICU, before being transferred to a specialist acquired brain injury inpatient rehabilitation unit for four weeks. Total duration of post-traumatic amnesia was 30 days. During his inpatient stay, he was noted to be verbose and tangential in conversation, becoming fixated on specific topics. He was also observed to make inappropriate comments to female staff about their appearance.

Cognitive assessment. Brief neuropsychological assessment during Shane's inpatient admission (five weeks post-injury) revealed attentional variability, slowed speed of information processing and pronounced executive deficits including difficulty with self-monitoring, verbal reasoning, shifting set and mental flexibility. On repeat neuropsychological assessment 8 months post-injury, while there was evidence of some improvement in cognitive functioning, Shane demonstrated ongoing mild to moderate reductions in attention, processing speed and executive functioning (reasoning, problem-solving, self-monitoring, inhibition and flexible thinking).

Social and occupational functioning post-discharge. On discharge, Shane had no residual physical impairments. However, he was not medically cleared to drive or return to work due to his cognitive difficulties. Shane had minimal insight into the extent of his cognitive changes or their impact on his day-to-day functioning. During the first few months post-discharge, he spent most of his time at home. His family took over the daily operations and financial management of the business. Shane expressed frustration and resentment towards his family for keeping him 'trapped' and 'on a leash'. When he did attend social events, Shane's wife reported that he was 'blunt' in his interpersonal style and would say inappropriate and hurtful things to family and friends. He was also noted to have difficulty regulating his emotions, including managing anger. He did not appear to notice the impact that this had on his relationships.

In response to concerns raised by Shane's wife, he was referred to a specialist brain injury behaviour management programme. This intervention initially focused on supporting Shane's wife, including providing her with education about his behaviour and cognitive changes, possible triggers for his behaviours and appropriate management strategies. Shane was subsequently referred to outpatient neuropsychology for ongoing management and support. He attended regular therapy sessions with a neuropsychologist, which focused on learning strategies to support his cognitive deficits and psychological interventions such as relaxation for managing stress.

After 6 months, Shane returned to work in a limited capacity. This involved accompanying his daughter to the business site, where he would sit and observe the day's activities. Initially, Shane reported feeling frustrated that even though he was back at work, he still wasn't allowed to run his own business. However, he soon realised that being back at work was exhausting, even in this limited capacity. With time, and with ongoing support from his treating neuropsychologist, Shane expressed less frustration with his family and the perceived restrictions on his life. His family reported that his mood was improved, and he gradually became more appropriate in his interactions with others. Though he was not able to return to his previous level of occupational functioning, he came to enjoy his new role and the sense of purpose and routine of attending work each day.

The expected clinical course of cognitive recovery after TBI is one of gradual improvement. In cases of mild TBI, where there is only a transient alteration of consciousness, any cognitive difficulties usually recover to baseline levels within the first few weeks or months post-injury.[51–54] Moderate and severe TBI is associated with more pronounced cognitive impairment, with the most spontaneous improvement likely during the first 6 to 12 months post-injury when neuroplastic changes can facilitate some restoration of cognitive function.[55, 56] This tends to reach a plateau at around 2 years.[57, 58] While some gradual ongoing improvement after this time is possible, studies of long-term follow-up have found cognitive difficulties can persist beyond 10 years post-injury.[59]

Secondary Cognitive Consequences of TBI

In addition to the primary effects of a TBI on cognitive functioning, diverse neurological, psychological and psychosocial sequelae of a TBI can further undermine cognitive integrity.

Mood

TBI is associated with an increased risk of mood and anxiety disorders.[60] Meta-analytic findings indicate that between 27% and 38% of adults with TBI develop clinically significant symptoms of depression,[61] and 37% develop anxiety disorders.[62–64] Aetiology is likely multifactorial, including neurobiological factors (i.e. susceptibility of frontal and limbic regions to traumatic injury), psychological factors (i.e. adjustment to the impact of the injury) and psychosocial factors (i.e. social support).[65, 66] A pre-injury history of mental health disorder increases the risk for the development of mood and anxiety disorders after TBI.[67, 68]

Symptoms of mood disturbance and anxiety are independently associated with cognitive difficulties in healthy and clinical populations, particularly affecting the same domains of attention, memory, information processing speed and executive function.[69–72] Thus, in the setting of TBI, emotional comorbidities can magnify the primary cognitive effects of the brain injury, leading to more pronounced and disabling symptoms.[68] Critically, however, these secondary cognitive consequences are potentially reversible, with emerging evidence that cognitive problems associated with low mood and anxiety may be remediated with treatment in healthy adults[73] and in TBI specifically.[74] Thus, careful monitoring of mood is recommended to facilitate early detection and treatment of potential mood disturbance after TBI.

Fatigue

Fatigue is common after brain injury, with prevalence estimates ranging from 30% to 70%.[75] The experience of fatigue after TBI can be both cognitive and physical and can affect individuals across the spectrum of injury severity from mild to severe.[76, 77] Individuals with TBI may describe it as 'hitting a wall', beyond which they can no longer engage in continued cognitive or physical effort.[78] This can be particularly pronounced following sensory stimulation or prolonged engagement in cognitive tasks.[79] Post-TBI fatigue is commonly cited as a significant barrier to returning to valued activities in the community and can have a major impact on quality of life.[41] It can also be chronic, persisting for many years post-injury.[80, 81]

In terms of mechanisms, it has been proposed that the effort required to compensate for slowed processing speed and attentional problems to achieve an adequate level of function in day-to-day life is a significant contributor to fatigue after TBI.[75] This is supported by findings from empirical studies of subjective fatigue and cognitive performance.[82, 83] Additionally, functional MRI studies have shown that, compared to healthy controls, individuals with TBI demonstrate increased activation in task-related brain regions while performing a cognitive task, suggestive of increased cerebral effort required to complete the task.[84] The relationship between fatigue and cognition is reciprocal, with cognitive difficulties not only contributing to this picture, but being further exacerbated by fatigue. In particular, greater subjective cognitive fatigue after TBI is associated with slower processing speed and more errors on tasks of complex attention.[75, 85–87] Fatigue also interacts with other common sequelae of TBI, including sleep disturbance, pain, depression and anxiety.[88, 89] As such, timely and appropriate management of these conditions is important.

Primary Cognitive Sequelae of Epilepsy

The peak global body for epilepsy care and research, the International League Against Epilepsy, defines epilepsy as a disease whose hypersynchronous electrical activity entrains and is propagated along the networks that organise the brain.[90] This leads to both paroxysmal disruption of networks specialised for neurocognitive processing, as well as chronic abnormalities in the topography, structure and functioning of these same networks stemming from interictal epileptic discharges and epilepsy-related pathologies.[7,8,91–94] Some degree of cognitive impairment can thus be detected in many people with epilepsy,[95] and cognitive comorbidities are now considered to be an intrinsic feature of the disease.[96] Cognitive comorbidities are a major economic and psychological burden on people with epilepsy, with self-report ratings indicating that cognitive deficits significantly reduce day-to-day functioning and quality of life, and may limit employability.[97]

Research focusing on delineating the clinical factors that contribute to the development of cognitive dysfunction in people with epilepsy variously emphasise the deleterious role of seizure frequency and severity, frequency of subclinical interictal epileptiform activity, seizure-induced head strikes, long duration of epilepsy and the age at onset of seizures.[5, 98] The influence of the latter, however, is nuanced. In childhood-onset disease, epileptiform activity and gross brain pathology can skew the normal development of cognitive networks, resulting in either impaired cognitive function or the transfer of cognitive hubs proximal to the seizure focus to intact regions of the brain.[99] The development of seizures in adult-onset epilepsy can not only lead to focalised impairments equivalent to those seen in childhood-onset cases when they are associated with brain pathology or depression,[100] but may also accelerate senility due to the 'double hit' of aging on cognitive networks already compromised by epilepsy.[101]

More broadly, cognitive impairments in people with epilepsy have been conceptualised as an intrinsic feature of the underlying network disease; that is, the disease process that gives rise to seizures also gives rise to cognitive impairment.[102] Supporting this, severe memory impairments in focal epilepsy patients with no MRI-resolvable brain lesion can be similar to those in patients with gross pathology, like hippocampal sclerosis or tumours.[103] Moreover, the finding that cognitive impairments may be evident in untreated patients with newly diagnosed seizures[104, 105] suggests that the disease can disrupt the healthy development of cognitive networks in the absence of overt seizures. This means that abnormal neurocognitive function in epilepsy may not be purely a consequence of damage secondary to seizures and pathology, as was traditionally believed.

Epilepsy can arise from any region of the cerebrum or cerebellum, and therefore all cognitive domains and networks are vulnerable in this population (see Helmstaedter et al., 2011 for a review[95]). Some cognitive deficits in epilepsy are markers of large-scale network compromise taking the form of slowed information processing speed (bradyphrenia) and attentional inefficiency, which are seen across many focal and generalised epilepsy syndromes but are especially pronounced in drug-resistant cases.[95] In contrast, circumscribed, focal seizure onsets are classically associated with cognitive features attributable to dysfunction in the onset zone. For example, memory disorder in temporal lobe epilepsy (see Saling, 2009 for a review[106]), executive dysfunction in frontal lobe epilepsy,[107–109] and language symptoms such as dysnomia or paraphasias in people with disease localised to the language-dominant hemisphere.[110] Given the day-to-day personal relevance of social cognitive deficits, there is also growing evidence that relative to healthy controls both focal and generalised forms of epilepsy can be associated with deficits in theory of mind and facial emotion recognition,[111, 112] with reduced social cognition linked to an earlier age at seizure onset.[112]

Secondary Cognitive Consequences of Epilepsy

In addition to the disturbance to neurocognitive networks by seizures and the underlying disease, people with epilepsy can also contend with various medical, psychological and psychosocial sequelae of their illness that can secondarily undermine cognitive efficiency.

Unipolar depression is the most common psychiatric symptom of epilepsy, with up to 50% of patients developing a clinically significant mood disorder at some point in their lifetime.[113, 114] Symptom profiling of depression in epilepsy reveals a predominant phenotype (base rate = 17%) taking the form of a Cognitive Depression that is characterised by cognitive symptoms of depression and dysphoria. Epilepsy patients with cognitive depression also have prominent memory deficits relative to nondepressed patients or those with a somatic or vegetative phenotype of depression in epilepsy (base rate = 7%).[114] Reduced new learning and delayed recall is more prominent in epilepsy patients with major depression, especially in patients with left temporal foci,[115–117] with severity of depressive symptoms able to predict the scope of the memory dysfunction.[118] This laterality effect has been interpreted as reflecting the depletion of cognitive reserve in people with depression exacerbating already poor verbal elaboration skills. After epilepsy surgery, temporal lobe epilepsy patients with clinically elevated depressive symptoms evidence greater verbal memory decline than nondepressed patients,[119] while frontal lobe epilepsy patients with elevated depressive symptoms show greater reductions in cognitive control.[120] These poor cognitive outcomes cannot be accounted for by differences in seizure outcome or post-operative mood alone, and they predict cognitive outcome beyond what can be achieved with pre-surgical memory indices. This may indicate that cognitive function after epilepsy surgery is more vulnerable in the context of depression, with the nature of the cognitive impairment shaped by the underlying focalisation of the patient's epilepsy syndrome. Further research, however, is needed to determine whether these cognitive 'declines' are reversed when a patient's psychiatric state improves.

The **surgical and medical treatment of seizures** can also lead to cognitive disorder. For the 30% of patients whose seizures are drug-resistant, epilepsy surgery offers the best chance of seizure freedom.[121] For some patients, however, this opportunity costs them a decline in their cognitive function.[122] In their review of 474 cases in the epilepsy programme at Queen's Square, London, Baxendale and Thompson[122] identified that nearly 40% of patients who underwent epilepsy surgery experienced a decline in their memory function, while 12% suffered a 'double hit' of cognitive decrement occurring in the context of ongoing post-surgical seizures. Initial longitudinal evidence suggests that when surgery does result in seizure freedom over the long term, memory function can recover to baseline levels, with drug load reduction specifically linked to improvements in executive functions.[123] Notably, this latter study of 161 German patients did not find evidence for accelerated cognitive decline in the years after surgery over the long term. Chapter 13 of this book specifically details the **iatrogenic impact of antiepileptic medications** on cognition, with sedation and bradyphrenia common side effects.

Cognitive Profile of Post-traumatic Epilepsy

Post-traumatic Epilepsy: a 'Double Hit' to Cognition?

There is a paucity of empirical research that directly investigates the cognitive sequelae of PTE in humans.[124, 125] However, given the above findings of elevated rates of cognitive deficits in both epilepsy and TBI, it is conceivable that PTE may serve to exacerbate the existing cognitive problems resulting from TBI alone and result in a 'double hit' to cognitive function.

Early work by Dikmen & Reitan (1978)[126] explored whether the cognitive sequelae of PTE were attributable to structural neurological damage rather than the epilepsy per se. They did this by comparing the normal cognitive functioning of healthy controls ($n = 20$) to that of two subgroups of head-injured patients: one with PTE and persistent focal neurological signs (n=22) and the other with PTE uncomplicated by neurological findings (n=27). Their cross-sectional study revealed that both PTE groups showed equivalently poor cognitive functioning relative to healthy controls, suggesting that the epileptic activity associated with PTE underpins its poor cognitive outcomes rather than gross brain pathology.

More recently, to explore the 'double hit' hypothesis, Semple and colleagues (2019)[4] reviewed both clinical and preclinical evidence pertaining to emotional, cognitive and psychosocial outcomes after PTE. Their review identified only a small handful of studies that had empirically investigated cognitive function in a cohort of people with PTE. Of these, two failed to find any evidence to support the notion that individuals with PTE experienced worse cognitive outcomes than TBI patients without seizures, after accounting for severity of TBI (N = 143 and 210)[125, 127] In contrast, a longitudinal study by Raymont *et al.* (2010)[128] assessing the cognitive outcomes of 199 Vietnam War veterans with penetrating head injuries found that PTE was predictive of a significantly greater decline in intelligence scores from pre-injury to 35-years post-injury, even when accounting for pre-injury intelligence scores and brain volume loss. Furthermore, duration of PTE was predictive of decline in intelligence scores between phase 2 to 3 of the study (i.e., between 15- and 35-years post-injury). Their findings suggest that PTE may have a cumulative, deleterious impact on general cognitive function relative to TBI alone, and it may predispose individuals to a more rapid cognitive decline later in life.[128]

Together, these limited studies provide tentative evidence for the hypothesis that people with PTE may be vulnerable to experiencing a 'double hit' to their cognition relative to people with TBI alone, although the nature and severity of their deficits relative to people with epilepsy alone remains to be clarified. More striking is the lack of extant literature, highlighting the vast gap in our existing knowledge of cognitive outcomes in PTE. Further research that systematically investigates the neuropsychological sequelae of PTE relative to both neurological populations (e.g. TBI/epilepsy) as well as healthy controls is urgently needed before stronger conclusions can be drawn.

Principles of Neuropsychological Rehabilitation for PTE

This section seeks to provide a model of cognitive rehabilitation for PTE, taking into account the secondary features of the disorder that can additionally undermine cognitive efficiency such as fatigue, sedation, depression and psychosocial restrictions. A barrier to this endeavour, however, is that there is little research into optimising cognitive rehabilitation for people with epilepsy[129] and seemingly none specific to people with PTE. This is a reasonable gap in the literature given there is limited evidence to date that PTE represents a distinct neurocognitive syndrome from TBI and/or epilepsy alone, with the nature of deficits similar but potentially just more severe in the combined form. As such we base this model on the well-established principles of neuropsychological rehabilitation for TBI and adapt it to account for the issues specific to comorbid epilepsy where scientific evidence allows.

Neuropsychological rehabilitation in PTE is an interactive process between the patient, family, community and health care team.[132] It seeks to optimise the functional capabilities of people who have cognitive or behavioural limitations resulting from the TBI and/or epilepsy, for which there is no known cure. It does not emphasise full restoration of function to premorbid levels; instead it seeks to maximise patient and family quality of life despite the patient's cognitive and behavioural limitations[130] by optimising independence and participation in the community. It achieves these aims through the use of medications, activity modifications, physical therapy, cognitive retraining, assistive devices and compensatory strategies, as well as adjunctive experiential therapy approaches involving art, animal care, music and drama.[131]

Remediating cognitive limitations can also be essential to patients achieving their goals with other health disciplines during the rehabilitation process. This necessitates a holistic approach to rehabilitation incorporating multi- or inter-disciplinary teamwork (see 'Freya' below).[129] Holistic rehabilitation of cognitive impairments aims to (i) sensitively increase

Case Vignette 8.2: 'Freya' The role of interdisciplinary teamwork in the rehabilitation setting

Freya is a 44-year-old female who developed PTE a few weeks after sustaining a moderate TBI in a cycling race. She currently has a generalised tonic-clonic seizure around once every 8 weeks despite pharmacotherapy with sodium valproate. She also incurred numerous lower limb orthopaedic injuries in her accident, and her rehabilitation goal is to return to a much-loved pastime of jogging. Specifically, she aims to build up to a 5-kilometre jog without stopping over the coming 6 months.

Freya's capability to achieve this physical goal is currently undermined by her cognitive difficulties. She is finding it hard to concentrate and follow instructions in her physiotherapy sessions, and secondary to some attentional impairments, she has trouble remembering the at-home exercises prescribed by the physiotherapist. This means Freya is not making as much physical progress as she had hoped. Freya has also identified an emotional barrier to achieving her goal; namely, she is scared of having a seizure whilst out jogging in the community and 'being taken advantage of' by an opportunistic sexual predator.

To assist Freya, the neuropsychologist is working collaboratively with Freya and her physiotherapist to develop tailored compensatory and environmental strategies to circumvent her attentional difficulties in her physio sessions, to allow her to physically achieve her goal. This includes reducing distractions by shifting her sessions to a quieter time of day, as well as writing down all instructions relevant to her at-home programme. The neuropsychologist is also working therapeutically with Freya to identify cognitive and behavioural strategies for her seizure-related anxiety, including systematic desensitisation of her 'nightmare scenario' and organising a roster of friends and family to accompany her as she builds up her jogging confidence.

patient awareness of their acquired limitations; (ii) work with the patient and support network to develop compensatory skills tailored to each individual's cognitive profile of strengths and weaknesses; (iii) provide psychoeducation, cognitive and social skills retraining and therapeutic interventions to minimise the impact of the patient's deficits; and (iv) support family members and other carers to reduce burnout.[131] The success of this endeavour broadly depends on effective goal setting, addressing the emotional sequelae of PTE, designing appropriate cognitive strategies, as well as recognising and managing the psychosocial barriers to rehabilitation that are specific to TBI and epilepsy.[132, 133]

Goal-focused. A cornerstone of cognitive rehabilitation with any patient population is the development of 'SMART' goals from the outset of patient engagement.[131]

SMART goals are:

- *Specific*: describe exactly what the patient wants to be able to do, in their own words;
- *Measurable*: decide how you will know when the goal is met. This may require setting multiple sub-goals in order to reach the major goal;
- *Achievable*: is this a realistic endeavour?
- *Relevant*: is this goal important to the patient and his/her values?
- *Timely*: decide in what time frame the goal will be achieved.

In the second Case Vignette of Freya, her SMART goal is to return to jogging (S); namely to be able to jog for 5 kilometres non-stop (M). This is deemed (A)chievable given her prognosis for physical recovery and her premorbid aptitude for the same activity, and it is an endeavour that brings her a sense of mindfulness and achievement (R). Finally, Freya hopes to attain this goal in 6 months (T).

The collaboration between the patient, team and support network in delineating rehabilitation goals is essential in empowering patients to take control of their own disability and to ensure that the goals set are relevant to the life they want to live. Amongst the health care team, a multidisciplinary approach is emphasised to co-ordinate the rehabilitation goals of patients.[129] In the case of Freya, interventions designed to compensate for her cognitive impairments were a key element in achieving her specific goal with physiotherapy to improve her lower limb function sufficiently to be able to jog a medium distance. It is also important for the patient and carers to identify potential barriers to achieving goals, such as financial barriers, cognitive or physical disability or lack of transport.

Cognitive Strategies

Prior to implementation of specific cognitive strategies, a comprehensive neuropsychological assessment is recommended. By integrating data from a range of sources, including performance on formal cognitive tasks, interviews with the patient and informant, measures of day-to-day functioning and behavioural observations, this assessment can be used to build a comprehensive profile of the individual's cognitive strengths and weaknesses. It is important to consider the person's strengths and skills, how the cognitive deficits are manifesting in everyday life, the day-to-day cognitive demands placed on the person and specific goals (as outlined in the section above) when selecting strategies for cognitive rehabilitation. In the absence of literature investigating the efficacy of cognitive strategies in PTE, the following sections draw upon the most up-to-date evidence-based practice recommendations available for cognitive rehabilitation after brain injury.

Attention and Processing Speed

Evidence from a recent systematic review[134] and recommendations from an international panel of experts (INCOG)[135] support the use of metacognitive strategy training for addressing problems with attention and information processing on everyday functional tasks, particularly for deficits in the mild to moderate range.[134, 135] This includes simple strategies, such as breaking information down into smaller, meaningful 'chunks', as well as formal training approaches such as Time Pressure Management (TPM) strategy training, developed by Fasotti and colleagues.[136] TPM aims to increase the individual's awareness of the effects of slowed processing speed and supports the use of self-instructional techniques or other steps to reduce time pressure (e.g. asking a person to repeat themselves, or recording information and playing it back later). Evidence from a randomised control trial (RCT) supports the use of this approach for improving coping with slowed information processing.[136]

There is also evidence from RCTs to support the use of cognitive training on dual tasks of attention, with improvements most likely on tasks similar to those trained.[134, 135] Environmental modifications that aim to reduce task attentional demands and maximise functioning (e.g. minimising distractions in the environment or using prompts to shift attention to another component of the task) are also frequently used in clinical practice.[137] However, more research evidence is required to support these recommendations.[135] The *sole* use of computer-based programs for improving attention and working memory is not recommended, due to findings of a lack of generalisation beyond the trained tasks to everyday functioning.[134, 138] Rather, this may be considered one part of a comprehensive rehabilitation program delivered under the guidance of a clinical neuropsychologist to build awareness and support the generalisation of learnings.[134]

Memory

Compensatory memory strategies aim to maximise the individual's everyday function via internal or external strategies. Internal strategies require conscious effort to improve memory encoding, for example, by grouping a shopping list into different semantic categories, such as fruit, vegetables and meat.[139] External strategies are those that rely on support beyond the self, and these include the use of diaries, notebooks, smartphones and whiteboards. There is good quality evidence for the effectiveness of internal and external strategy instruction in the rehabilitation of memory impairments after TBI.[134] For effective implementation, internal strategies require the person to have a degree of intact executive function and self-awareness, and thus they tend to be more effective for mild to moderate memory problems.[134, 140] Individuals with severe memory impairment after TBI typically benefit more from external supports and reminders, particularly when there is a support person available to prompt the use of these aids.[141] In choosing the most appropriate external memory aid, consideration should be given to the person's age, prior experience with technology, premorbid use of memory devices, cognitive profile and any physical comorbidities.[134, 141] Overall, compensatory memory strategies that align closely with a person's everyday tasks and activities are most likely to be used and therefore be successful.[142]

Executive Function

Metacognitive strategy training is recommended as a practice standard for addressing problems with executive function amongst adults with brain injury, based on evidence from several systematic reviews and meta-analyses.[134,143–146] Metacognitive instructive techniques are particularly recommended for addressing problems with planning, organization and problem-solving, with an emphasis on targeting improvement on everyday functional tasks.[143] Interventions are typically multifaceted, including components such as goal setting, goal management training, time pressure management, self-monitoring and direct feedback.[147] Direct feedback interventions, which seek to build the person's awareness and self-regulation skills through verbal, visual and/or experiential feedback, have been shown to be particularly useful for improving self-awareness of deficits after brain injury.[148–150]

There is also evidence to support the use of strategies promoting the analysis, assimilation and synthesis of complex material for improving reasoning skills after brain injury.[134, 143] For example, in an RCT of their Strategic Memory and Reasoning Training (SMART) Group programme, Vas and colleagues[151] trained adults with TBI to use a range of strategies, including filtering, focusing and chunking, linking, zooming and generalising, to extract meaning from complex material such as movies and news reports. This 12-session intervention resulted in significant improvements in reasoning, working memory and community participation, which were maintained 6 months post-completion of the programme. These interventions are less effective for individuals with severe cognitive impairment, however, as they require the individual to have sufficient self-awareness to identify the need for a strategy.[143] For those with pronounced impairments, additional environmental supports and structure in the way of external aids and prompts are recommended.

Social Cognition

Social cognition has emerged more recently as a target for treatment after brain injury. In a recent systematic review, Vallat-Azouvi and colleagues[152] identified 16 studies reporting treatment for social cognitive deficits after TBI, of which nine were RCTs. The majority of studies to date have examined the efficacy of specific training programmes to improve facial affect recognition, with mixed but promising results.[153–156] These interventions typically encourage the person to attend to areas of the face involved in emotional expression via verbal prompts, computer programs or video-based observation and instruction. Findings of the efficacy of interventions addressing other specific aspects of social cognition, such as theory of mind, have also been mixed.[157] These treatments aim to improve the individual's ability to infer what another person is thinking or feeling through the use of stories, cartoons, picture series, videos or role plays. There is some evidence for treatments targeting emotion regulation after TBI. For example, Aboulafia-Brakha and Ptak[158] found that a group anger management intervention could increase the use of coping strategies and reduce anger levels.

Combined treatment approaches that target multiple domains of social cognition have shown the most promising findings.[159] For example, Westerhof-Evers and colleagues[160] developed a multifaceted treatment for impairments in social cognition and emotion regulation (T-ScEmo) that includes compensatory strategies to improve emotion recognition, theory of mind and social skills, delivered in weekly 1-hour sessions for 16–20 weeks. The findings from this RCT showed that, when compared to a computerised cognitive training program, T-ScEmo resulted in significant improvements on tests of emotion recognition and theory of mind, ratings of empathic behaviour and participation in society for individuals with TBI, and these gains were maintained at 5-month follow-up.

Overall, although this field is still in its infancy, there are encouraging findings of the efficacy of some treatment approaches. Given problems with low sample sizes and inconsistent findings regarding generalisation to everyday functioning, further high quality studies are needed. Treatment programmes that hold most promise for generalisation of skills to day-to-day functioning are those that have an experiential basis, take a collaborative approach and are contextualised.[161]

Addressing Emotional Comorbidities to Achieve Cognitive Goals

As outlined earlier, depression and anxiety are highly prevalent and can contribute to cognitive deficits and reduced quality of life in PTE.[162] Individuals with PTE report that seizures have a negative impact on their ability to cope with the effects of the brain injury and act as a barrier to engaging in social activities in the community, which may further undermine emotional and cognitive functioning.[163] As such, a comprehensive and multidisciplinary approach to cognitive rehabilitation in PTE should include assessment and management of any emotional comorbidities.

Unfortunately, there is little research examining the efficacy of psychological approaches for addressing emotional disturbance in PTE. However, there are psychological treatments that have been found to be effective in TBI and epilepsy, and thus may hold promise for PTE. Cognitive behaviour therapy (CBT) is an extensively researched and well-validated psychological treatment for anxiety and depression in the general population.[164] CBT is a short-term, goal-oriented, structured form of psychotherapy that can be adapted to suit the needs of individuals with specific health conditions.[165] A modified CBT approach has been found to be effective in reducing symptoms of depression and anxiety after TBI.[166]

For the patient with PTE, a CBT programme incorporating tailored, neurobiologically informed psychoeducation on the emotional and cognitive consequences of brain injury and seizures may help to frame and normalise some of the challenges. Practical modifications to accommodate for cognitive impairments include scheduling shorter therapy sessions and frequent rest breaks, ensuring repetition of key information, providing written summaries to support learning, using concrete examples to explain abstract concepts and using external memory aids such as smartphone reminders to support the completion of homework tasks or session attendance.[167, 168] Psychological interventions also need to be sensitive to the ongoing challenges associated with PTE, including careful management of risk factors, activity limitations associated with seizures and the impact of anti-epileptic drug treatments.

TBI-specific Considerations for Rehabilitation

TBI has been described as a 'silent' or 'hidden' disability. Although many individuals with TBI have no physically discernible sign of disability, they can experience cognitive, social and emotional deficits that act as a major barrier to successful participation in the community, as highlighted throughout this chapter.[169–171] Misconceptions about TBI have been reported amongst the general public and by some health professionals.[172, 173] There is an expectation that a person who appears 'normal' should behave normally, and so family, friends and work colleagues may overestimate the abilities of brain-injured individuals with no overt physical signs of disability.[174] The degree of visibility of injury can impact on attributions of behaviour: when there is no visible marker of disability, the individual's actions (e.g. behaving in a way that is socially inappropriate) are more likely to be perceived as intentional rather than attributed to a neurological impairment.[175, 176]

The stigmatising and prejudicial attitudes held by the general public about individuals with TBI, particularly those with no overt signs of disability, may interfere with rehabilitation efforts.[177, 178] In PTE, this is compounded by the stigma associated with epilepsy, as discussed in the section below. Minimisation, trivialisation or misattribution of an individual's cognitive deficits can invalidate the person's experience and may undermine recovery. For this reason, it is important for clinicians to be aware of the diversity of cognitive, emotional and behavioural sequelae in PTE, and the significant impact that these symptoms can have on the person's everyday life, including the ability to work, study and maintain relationships. From the perspectives of the person with brain injury and the family, it is the emotional and behavioural symptoms that appear to have the greatest impact on the quality of life and the family's caring burden over the long term.[179]

One of the most common and disabling 'hidden' symptoms of TBI is fatigue. As discussed earlier in this chapter, fatigue can interact with and exacerbate primary cognitive difficulties following brain injury. In PTE, poorly managed fatigue may also represent a risk factor for reduced seizure control. Thus, improved management of fatigue may represent both a target for rehabilitation and an important consideration when structuring a rehabilitation programme for a patient with PTE.

Behavioural management techniques can help the individual to manage cognitive fatigue and minimise its effects on day-to-day life. First, the rehabilitation clinician might work together with the person with PTE to monitor and record fluctuations in fatigue levels over the course of a week. By revealing patterns in fatigue levels, including changes in response to specific activities or times of day, this exercise can provide valuable information to guide subsequent interventions. Strategies can then be tailored to the individual and may include, for example, scheduling activities for the time of the day when the person typically feel at his/her best, taking frequent breaks, keeping therapy sessions brief, delegating tasks to others, engaging in one task after another rather than multi-tasking, minimising stimulation in the environment and implementing healthy sleeping habits (e.g. regular bedtime routine, minimising naps during the day).[78, 180]

These behavioural management strategies can be complemented by more structured psychological interventions, which have been found to be effective in treating fatigue after TBI and may hold promise in PTE. For example, an RCT of patients with TBI or stroke found that an 8-week programme of mindfulness-based stress reduction resulted in improvements in mental fatigue and cognitive performance.[181] More recently, in an RCT conducted by Nguyen and colleagues[182] an eight-session adapted CBT programme was found to improve sleep quality, daily fatigue levels and depression symptoms amongst adults with TBI.

Epilepsy-specific Considerations for Rehabilitation

Although they are paroxysmal in duration, the sudden and often unearthly looking nature of epileptic seizures has for millennia distressed those who witness them and alienated their sufferers. Until relatively recently people with epilepsy were largely condemned by society as insane, intellectually stunted or possessed by evil spirits, connotations that persist in some regional and religious cultures.[183] While on balance the increasing recognition of epilepsy as a medical illness to be viewed empathetically has improved social acceptance for people with the disease, some continue to experience both felt and enacted stigma that, in part, stems from a lack of familiarity with epilepsy in the general community.[184] *Felt stigma* refers to feelings of shame and expectation of discrimination internalised by people with epilepsy, which prevents them from disclosing their illness in fear of social alienation and the withdrawal of opportunities. More overtly, *enacted stigma* takes the form of unfair treatment by others on the basis of the person's epilepsy; this includes being passed over for vocational advancement, deprived of educational opportunities and bullying or shunning. During the rehabilitation process, clinicians need to be mindful of both the patient's internalised stigma as well as potential societal attitudes towards epilepsy that might prove to be barriers to goal advancement.[185] For instance, a person with PTE may be unwilling to disclose their seizure status to an employer during return-to-work planning, due to either valid or exaggerated fears of being reassigned to other duties or dismissed. In cases where failure to disclose epilepsy poses an unacceptable safety risk to the patient or the community (e.g. a high-rise window cleaner, roofer) the clinician must balance ethical considerations around confidentiality and public safety and look for opportunities to support individuals to disclose this information on their own terms. This may involve problem-solving, cognitive therapeutic techniques, providing psychoeducation to a workplace and bureaucratic support in the case of unemployment.

Another consideration when collaboratively planning rehabilitation strategies around epilepsy is that many such individuals are unable to drive. This is rated by many patients as their chief bugbear in living with epilepsy.[186] Not being able to drive constitutes a major loss of independence for many adults, particularly those who must then rely upon others to take them to work, appointments, social engagements, etc. Such arrangements can make people with epilepsy feel like a burden upon others and exacerbate feelings of poor self-worth, discouraging them from asking for help and in some cases leading to social isolation. Overcoming these barriers may involve public transport training or perhaps cognitive therapies to challenge patient beliefs about the magnitude to which they are a burden.

Future Directions

A detailed literature search by the current authors could find only five original observational studies examining the cognitive sequelae of PTE in humans. As such, the field calls for large-scale neuropsychological research comparing the cognitive functioning of a cohort of well-characterized PTE to matched samples of people with TBI alone and epilepsy alone, so that the nature and aetiology of any specific deficits associated with PTE can be delineated. While the enormous heterogeneity of both TBI and epilepsy adds complexity to this endeavour, empirical evidence around the trajectory of cognitive (dys)function will improve the accuracy of prognostic counselling for people with PTE and their families, to the benefit of patient rehabilitation and well-being.

Conclusions

In sum, damage incurred to the brain due to a TBI can lead to impairments in multiple cognitive functions, including attention, new learning and memory, speed of information processing, executive functions and social cognition. Similarly, people with epilepsy are vulnerable to a range of cognitive deficits that can have a pronounced impact on quality of life and psychosocial functioning. Although limited, studies have begun to formally examine cognition in PTE, with tentative evidence that the onset of seizures in the post-traumatic period may further undermine the integrity of already compromised neurocognitive systems, resulting in a 'double hit' to cognitive functioning. Given the diffuse damage associated with TBI, approaches to cognitive rehabilitation in PTE should be first guided by established models and research-evidence in TBI and adapted and extended to accommodate the limitations and specific needs of comorbid epilepsy. A holistic, team-based approach that seeks to optimise the patient's quality of life, independence and participation in the community despite cognitive and behavioural limitations is recommended.

Acknowledgements

The authors would like to thank Ms Jessamae Pieters for her assistance in preparing this chapter, specifically in undertaking a literature review and drafting text relevant to this review.

References

1. D.H. Lowenstein. Epilepsy after head injury: an overview. *Epilepsia* 2009;**50**:4–9.

2. L. Piccenna, G. Shears, T. O'Brien. Management of post-traumatic epilepsy: An evidence review over the last 5 years and future directions. *Epilepsia Open* 2017;**2**:123–44.

3. R.M. Verellen and J.E. Cavazos. Post-traumatic epilepsy: an overview. *Therapy* 2014;**7**:527–31.

4. B.D. Semple, A. Zamani, G. Rayner, *et al.* Affective, neurocognitive and psychosocial disorders associated with traumatic brain injury and post-traumatic epilepsy. *Neurobiol Dis* 2019;**123**:27–41.

5. G.L. Holmes and P.P. Lenck-Santini. Role of interictal epileptiform abnormalities in cognitive impairment. *Epilepsy Behav* 2006;**8**:504–15.

6. V. Dinkelacker, X. Xin, M. Baulac, *et al.* Interictal epileptic discharge correlates with global and frontal cognitive dysfunction in temporal lobe epilepsy. *Epilepsy Behav* 2016;**62**:197–203.

7. J.I. Stretton, G. Winston, M. Sidhu, *et al.* Neural correlates of working memory in temporal lobe epilepsy–an fMRI study. *NeuroImage* 2012;**60**:1696–703.

8. C. Tailby, G. Rayner, S.J. Wilson, *et al.* The spatiotemporal substrates of autobiographical recollection: Using event-related ICA to study cognitive networks in action. *NeuroImage* 2017;**152**:237–48.

9. M.L. Pearn, I.R. Niesman, J. Egawa, *et al.* Pathophysiology Associated with traumatic brain injury: Current treatments and potential novel therapeutics. *Cell Mol Neurobiol* 2017;**37**:571–85.

10. H.M. Bramlett and W.D. Dietrich. Long-term consequences of traumatic brain injury: Current status of potential mechanisms of injury and neurological outcomes. *J Neurotrauma* 2015;**32**:1834–8.

11. E.D. Bigler and E.D. Bigler. Anterior and middle cranial fossa in traumatic brain injury: Relevant neuroanatomy and neuropathology in the study of neuropsychological outcome. *Neuropsychol* 2007;**21**:515–31.

12. E. Fujiwara, M.L. Schwartz, F. Gao, *et al.* Ventral frontal cortex functions and quantified MRI in traumatic brain injury. *Neuropsychologia* 2008;**46**:461–74.

13. J.S. Beer, P.J. Oliver, D. Scabini, *et al.* Orbitofrontal cortex and social behavior: integrating self-monitoring and emotion-cognition interactions. *J Cogn Neurosci* 2006;**18**(6):871–9

14. M. Kringelbach. The human orbitofrontal cortex: linking reward to hedonic experience. *Nat Rev Neurosci* 2005;**6**:691–702.

15. J.M. Spikman, D.H. Boelen, G. H. Pijnenborg, *et al.* Who benefits from treatment for executive dysfunction after brain injury? Negative effects of emotion recognition deficits. *Neuropsychol Rehabil* 2013;**23**:824–45.

16. A.D. Moore and M. Stambrook. Cognitive moderators of outcome following traumatic brain injury: A conceptual model and implications for rehabilitation. *Brain Inj* 1995;**9**:109–30.

17. M.A. Struchen, A.N. Clark, A.M. Sander, *et al.* Relation of executive functioning and social communication measures to functional outcomes following traumatic brain injury. *NeuroRehabilitation* 2008;**23**:185–98.

18. T. Kay and S.M. Silver. The contribution of the neuropsychological evaluation to the vocational rehabilitation of the head-injured adult. *J Head Trauma Rehabil* 1988;**3**:65–76.

19. G. Spitz, J. Ponsford, D. Rudzki, *et al.* Association between cognitive performance and functional outcome following traumatic brain injury: A longitudinal multilevel examination. *Neuropsychol* 2012;**26**:604–12.

20. R.L. Wood and A. Worthington. Neurobehavioral abnormalities associated with executive dysfunction after traumatic brain injury. *Front Behav Neurosci* 2017;**11**:195.

21. R.C. Chan, D. Shum, T. Toulopoulou, *et al.* Assessment of executive functions: review of instruments and identification of critical issues. *Arch Clin Neuropsychol* 2008;**23**:201–16.

22. V.E. Johnson, W. Stewart, D.H. Smith. Axonal pathology in traumatic brain injury. *Exp Neurol*, 2013;**246**: 35–43.

23. G. Spitz, J.J. Maller, R. O'Sullivan, *et al.* White matter integrity following traumatic brain injury: The association with severity of injury and cognitive functioning. *Brain Topogr* 2013;**26**:648–60.

24. D. Sharp, G. Scott, R. Leech. Network dysfunction after traumatic brain injury. *Nat Rev Neurol* 2014;**10**:156–66.

25. M.M. van Eijck, G.G. Schoonman, J. van der Naalt, *et al.* Diffuse axonal injury after traumatic brain injury is a prognostic factor for functional outcome: a systematic review and meta-analysis, *Brain Inj* 2018;**32**:395–402.

26. J. Ponsford. Mechanism, recovery and sequelae of traumatic brain injury: A foundation for the REAL approach. In: Ponsford J., Sloan S., Snow P., eds. *Traumatic Brain Injury: Rehabilitation for Everyday Adaptive Living.* Hove, UK, Psychology Press, 2012;1–33.

27. D.R. Babbage, J. Yim, B. Zupan, *et al.* Meta-analysis of facial affect recognition difficulties after traumatic brain injury. *Neuropsychol* 2011;**25**:277–85.

28. S.R. Borgaro, G. Prigatano, C. Kwasnica, *et al.* Disturbances in affective communication following brain injury. *Brain Inj* 2004;**18**:33–9.

29. R.E.A. Green, G.R. Turner, W. F. Thompson. Deficits in facial emotion perception in adults with recent traumatic brain injury. *Neuropsychologia* 2004;**42**:133–41.

30. M. Ietswaart, M.V. Milders, J.R. Crawford, *et al.* Longitudinal aspects of emotion recognition in patients with traumatic brain injury. *Neuropsychologia* 2008;**46**:148–59.

31. S. McDonald, C. Bornhofen, C. Hunt. Addressing deficits in emotion recognition after severe traumatic brain injury: The role of focused attention and mimicry. *Neuropsychol Rehabil* 2009;**19**:321–39.

32. J.D. Henry, L.H. Phillips, J.R. Crawford, *et al.* Cognitive and psychosocial correlates of alexithymia following traumatic brain injury. *Neuropsychologia* 2006;**44**:62–72.

33. D. Neumann. Alexithymia after brain injury: What is it and why it deserves more attention. *Arch Phys Med Rehabil* 2013;**94**:e7.

34. C. Williams and R. Wood. Alexithymia and emotional empathy following traumatic brain injury. *J Clin Exp Neuropsychol* 2010;**32**:259–67.

35. M.V. Milders, S. Fuchs, J.R. Crawford. Neuropsychological impairments and changes in emotional and social behaviour following severe traumatic brain injury. *J Clin Exp Neuropsychol* 2003;**25**:157–72.

36. V. Havet-Thomassin, P. Allain, F. Etcharry-Bouyx, *et al.* What about theory of mind after severe brain injury? *Brain Inj* 2006;**20**:83–91.

37. J.F. Martin-Rodriguez, Leon-Carrion J. Theory of mind deficits in patients with acquired brain injury: a quantitative review. *Neuropsychologia* 2010;**48** (5):1181–91.

38. J.D. Henry, W. von Hippel, P. Molenberghs, *et al.* Clinical assessment of social cognitive function in neurological disorders. *Nat Rev Neurol* 2016;**12**:28.

39. M.H. Beauchamp and V. Anderson V. SOCIAL: An integrative framework for the development of social skills. *Psychol Bull* 2010;**136**:39–64.

40. M.R. Newsome, R.S. Scheibel, A.R. Mayer, *et al.* How functional connectivity between emotion regulation structures can be disrupted: Preliminary evidence from adolescents with moderate to severe traumatic brain injury. *J Int Neuropsychol Soc* 2013;**19**:911–24.

41. S. Palm, L. Rönnbäck, B. Johansson. Long-term mental fatigue after traumatic brain injury and impact on employment status. *J Rehab Med* 2017;**49**:228–33.

42. A. de Sousa, S. McDonald, J. Rushby, *et al.* Understanding deficits in empathy after traumatic brain injury: The role of affective responsivity. *Cortex* 2011;**47**:526–35.

43. R.L. Wood and C. Williams. Inability to empathize following traumatic brain injury. *J Int Neuropsychol Soc* 2008;**14**:289–96.

44. B. Caplan, J. Bogner, L. Brenner, *et al.* The relations of self-reported aggression to alexithymia, depression, and anxiety after traumatic brain injury. *J Head Trauma Rehabil* 2017;**32**:205–13.

45. K. Osborne-Crowley and S. McDonald, S. A review of social disinhibition after

traumatic brain injury. *J Neuropsychol* 2018;**12**:176–99.

46. C. Chesnel, C. Jourdan, E. Bayen, *et al.* Self-awareness four years after severe traumatic brain injury: discordance between the patient's and relative's complaints. Results from the PariS-TBI study. Clin *Rehab* 2018;**32**:692–704.

47. S. Lock, L. Jordan, K. Bryan, *et al.* Work after stroke: Focusing on barriers and enablers. *Disabil Soc* 2005;**20**:33–47.

48. M. Gosling and M. Oddy. Rearranged marriages: Marital relationships after head injury. *Brain Inj* 1999;**13**:785–96.

49. F. O'Keeffe, J. Dunne, M. Nolan, *et al.* 'The things that people can't see' The impact of TBI on relationships: an interpretative phenomenological analysis. *Brain Inj* 2020;**34**:496–507.

50. C.E. Salas, M. Casassus, L. Rowlands, *et al.* 'Relating through sameness': a qualitative study of friendship and social isolation in chronic traumatic brain injury, *Neuropsychol Rehabil* 2018;**28**:1161–78.

51. V.L. Feigin, A. Theadom, S. Barker-Collo, *et al.* Incidence of traumatic brain injury in New Zealand: A population-based study. *Lancet Neurol* 2003;**12**:53–64.

52. J.E. Karr, C.N. Areshenkoff, M.A. Garcia-Barrera. The neuropsychological outcomes of concussion: A systematic review of meta-analyses on the cognitive sequelae of mild traumatic brain injury. *Neuropsychol* 2014;**28**:321–36.

53. F. Tagliaferri, C. Compagnone, M. Korsic, *et al.* A systematic review of brain injury epidemiology in Europe. *Acta Neurochir (Wein)*, 2006;**148**:255–68.

54. M. McCrea, K.M. Guskiewicz, W. Marshall, *et al.* Acute effects and recovery time following concussion in collegiate football players: The NCAA concussion study. *JAMA* 2003;**290**:2556–63.

55. R. Teasell, N. Bayona, S. Marshall, *et al.* A systematic review of the rehabilitation of moderate to severe acquired brain injuries. *Brain Inj* 2007;**21**:107–12.

56. L. Turner-Stokes, A. Pick, A. Nair, *et al.* Multi-disciplinary rehabilitation for acquired brain injury in adults of working age. *Cochrane Database Syst Rev* 2005;**12**: Article No:CD004170.

57. S. Dikmen, J. Machamer, N. Temkin, *et al.* Neuropsychological recovery in patients with moderate to severe head injury: Two-year follow-up. *J Clin Exp Neuropsychol* 1990;**12**:507–19.

58. D. Schretlen and A.M. Shapiro. A quantitative review of the effects of traumatic brain injury on cognitive functioning. *Int Rev Psychiatry* 2003;**15**:341–9.

59. K. Draper and J.L. Ponsford. Cognitive functioning ten years following traumatic brain injury and rehabilitation. *Neuropsychol* 2008;**22**:618–25.

60. K. Gould, J. Ponsford, L. Johnston L, *et al.* Relationship between psychiatric disorders and 1-year psychosocial outcome following traumatic brain injury. *J Head Trauma Rehabil* 2011;**26**:79–89.

61. A.J. Osborn, J.L. Mathias, A. K. Fairweather-Schmidt. Depression following adult, non-penetrating traumatic brain injury: A meta-analysis examining methodological variables and sample characteristics. *Neurosci Biobehav Rev* 2014;**47**:1–15.

62. A.J. Osborn, J.L. Mathias, A. K. Fairweather-Schmidt, A. K. Prevalence of anxiety following adult traumatic brain injury: A meta-analysis comparing measures, samples and postinjury intervals. *Neuropsychol* 2016;**30**:247–61.

63. R.A. Bryant. Mental disorders and traumatic injury. *Depress Anxiety* 2011;**28**:99–102.

64. T. Hart, J.R. Fann, I. Chervoneva. Prevalence, risk factors, and correlates of anxiety at 1 year after moderate to severe traumatic brain injury. *Arch Phys Med Rehabil* 2016;**97**:701–7.

65. R.E. Jorge and S.E. Starkstein. Pathophysiologic aspects of major depression following traumatic brain injury. *J Head Trauma Rehabil* 2005;**20**:475–87.

66. S. Fleminger, D.L. Oliver, H.W. Williams, *et al.* The neuropsychiatry of depression after brain injury. *Neuropsychol Rehabil* 2003;**13(1–2)**:65–87.

67. S. Dikmen, C.H. Bombardier, J. Machamer J. Natural history of depression in traumatic brain injury. *Arch Phys Med Rehabil* 2004;**85**:1457–64.

68. R.E. Jorge, R.G. Robinson, D. Moser, *et al.* Major depression following traumatic brain injury. *Arch Gen Psychiatry* 2004;**61**:42–50.

69. R.S.C. Lee, D.F. Hermens, M.A. Porter, *et al.* A meta-analysis of cognitive deficits in first-episode Major Depressive Disorder. *J Affect Dis* 2010;**140**:113–24.

70. F. Ferreri, L.K. Lapp, Leann, C.S. Peretti. Current research on cognitive aspects of anxiety disorders. *Curr Opin Psychiatry* 2011;**24**:49–54.

71. H.R. Snyder. Major depressive disorder is associated with broad impairments on neuropsychological measures of executive function: A meta-analysis and review. *Psychol Bull* 2013;**139**:81–132.

72. H.R. Snyder, A. Miyake, B.L. Hankin. Advancing understanding of executive function impairments and psychopathology: Bridging the gap between clinical and cognitive approaches. *Front Psychol* 2015;**6**:328.

73. M. Butters, R. Bhalla, C. Andreescu, *et al.* Changes in neuropsychological functioning following treatment for late-life generalised anxiety disorder. *Br J Psychiatry* 2011;**199**:211–18.

74. J.R. Fann, J.M. Uomoto, W.J. Katon. Cognitive improvement with treatment of depression following mild traumatic brain injury. *Psychosomatics* 2001;**42**:48–54

75. A. Belmont, N. Agar, P. Azouvi. Subjective fatigue, mental effort, and attention deficits after severe traumatic brain injury. *Neurorehabil Neural Repair* 2009;**23**:939–44.

76. M.P. Dijkers and T. Bushnik. Assessing fatigue after traumatic brain injury: an evaluation of the Barroso Fatigue Scale. *J Head Trauma Rehabil* 2008;**23**:3–16.

77. C. Merritta, B. Cherian, A.S. Macaden, *et al.* Measurement of physical performance and objective fatigability in people with mild-to-moderate traumatic brain injury. *Int J Rehabil Res* 2010;**33**:109–14.

78. J.B. Cantor, W. Gordon, S. Gumber. What is post TBI fatigue? *NeuroRehabilitation* 2013;**32**:875–83.

79. B. Johansson and L. Ronnback. Evaluation of the Mental Fatigue Scale and its relation to cognitive and emotional functioning after traumatic brain injury or stroke. *Int J Phys Med Rehabil* 2014, 2:1.

80. T. Bushnik, J. Englander, J. Wright. Patterns of fatigue and its correlates over the first 2 years after traumatic brain injury. *J Head Trauma Rehabil* 2008;**23**:25–32.

81. M.A. Zumstein, M. Moser, M. Mottini, *et al.* Long-term outcome in patients with mild traumatic brain injury: A prospective observational study. *J Trauma* 2011;**71**:120–7.

82. T.A. Ashman, J.B. Cantor, W.A. Gordon. Objective measurement of fatigue following traumatic brain injury. *J Head Trauma Rehabil* 2008;**23**:33–40.

83. P. Azouvi, J. Couillet, M. Leclercq, *et al.* Divided attention and mental effort after severe traumatic brain injury. *Neuropsychologia* 2004;**42**:1260–8.

84. A.D. Kohl, G.R. Wylie, H.M. Genova, *et al.* The neural correlates of cognitive fatigue in traumatic brain injury using functional MRI. *Brain Inj* 2009;**23**:420–432.

85. B. Johansson, P. Berglund, L. Rönnbäck L. Mental fatigue and impaired information processing after mild and moderate traumatic brain injury. *Brain Inj* 2009;**23**:1027–40.

86. C. Ziino and J. Ponsford. Selective attention deficits and subjective fatigue following traumatic brain injury. *Neuropsychol* 2006;**20**:383–90.

87. C. Ziino and J. Ponsford. Vigilance and fatigue following traumatic brain injury. *J Int Neuropsychol Soc* 2006;**12**:100–10.

88. J.B. Cantor, T. Bushnik, K. Cicerone, *et al.* Insomnia, fatigue, and sleepiness in the

first 2 years after traumatic brain injury: an NIDRR TBI model system module study. *J Head Trauma Rehabil* 2012;27:E1–14.

89. J. Englander, T. Bushnik, J. Oggins, *et al.* Fatigue after traumatic brain injury: Association with neuroendocrine, sleep, depression and other factors. *Brain Inj* 2010;24:1379–88.

90. S.S. Spencer. Neural networks in human epilepsy: evidence of and implications for treatment. *Epilepsia* 2002;43:219–27.

91. D.N. Vaughan, G. Rayner, C. Tailby, *et al.* MRI-negative temporal lobe epilepsy: a network disorder of neocortical connectivity. *Neurol* 2016;87:1934–42.

92. M. Pedersen, A. Omidvarnia, E. K. Curwood, *et al.* The dynamics of functional connectivity in neocortical focal epilepsy. *NeuroImage Clin* 2017;15:209–14.

93. S.J. Wilson, D.F. Abbott, C. Tailby, *et al.* Changes in singing performance and fMRI activation following right temporal lobe surgery. *Cortex* 2013;49:2512–24.

94. F. Fahoum, R. Lopes, F. Pittau, *et al.* Widespread epileptic networks in focal epilepsies: EEG-fMRI study. *Epilepsia* 2012;53:1618–27.

95. C. Helmstaedter, B. Hermann, M. Lassonde, *et al.* eds. *Neuropsychology in the Care of People with Epilepsy.* France, John Libbey Eurotext, 2011.

96. I.E. Scheffer, S. Berkovic, G. Capovilla, *et al.* ILAE classification of the epilepsies: position paper of the ILAE Commission for Classification and Terminology. *Epilepsia* 2017;58:512–21.

97. G.A. Baker, J. Taylor, B. Hermann. How can cognitive status predispose to psychological impairment? *Epilepsy Behav* 2009;15:S31–5.

98. B. Korman, P. Krsek, M. Duchowny, *et al.* Early seizure onset and dysplastic lesion extent independently disrupt cognitive networks. *Neurol* 2013;81:745–51.

99. B.P. Hermann, M. Seidenberg, B. Bell. The neurodevelopmental impact of childhood onset temporal lobe epilepsy on brain structure and function and the risk of

progressive cognitive effects. *Prog Brain Res* 2002;135:429–38.

100. G. Rayner, G.D. Jackson, S.J. Wilson. Mechanisms of memory impairment in epilepsy depend on age at disease onset. *Neurol* 2016;87:1642–9.

101. L.E. Breuer, P. Boon, J.W. Bergmans, *et al.* Cognitive deterioration in adult epilepsy: does accelerated cognitive ageing exist? *Neurosci Biobehav Rev* 2016;64:1–11.

102. S.J. Wilson and S. Baxendale. The new approach to classification: rethinking cognition and behavior in epilepsy. *Epilepsy Behav* 2014;41:307–10.

103. G. Rayner, C. Tailby, G. Jackson G, *et al.* Looking beyond lesions for causes of neuropsychological impairment in epilepsy. *Neurol* 2019;92:e680–9.

104. J. Taylor, R. Kolamunnage-Dona, A. G. Marson, *et al.* Patients with epilepsy: cognitively compromised before start of antiepileptic drug treatment? *Epilepsia* 2010;51:48–56.

105. D. Tosun, K. Dabbs, R. Caplan, *et al.* Deformation-based morphometry of prospective neurodevelopmental changes in new onset paediatric epilepsy. *Brain* 2011;134:1003–14.

106. M.M. Saling. Verbal memory in mesial temporal lobe epilepsy: beyond material specificity. *Brain* 2009;132:570–82.

107. J.V. Baldo and A.P. Shimamura. Frontal lobes and memory. In: Baddely A.D., Kopelmann, M. D., Wilson B. A., eds. *The Handbook of Memory Disorders.* Hoboken, John Wiley & Sons Ltd, 2002.

108. J. O'Muircheartaigh and M. P. Richardson. Epilepsy and the frontal lobes. *Cortex* 2012;48:144–55.

109. G. Rayner, G.D. Jackson, S.J. Wilson. Behavioural profiles in frontal lobe epilepsy: autobiographic memory versus mood impairment. *Epilepsia* 2015;56:225–23.

110. M.J. Hamberger and W.T. Seidel. Auditory and visual naming tests: Normative and patients data for accuracy, response time, and tip-of-the-tongue. *J Int Neuropsychol Soc* 2003;9:479–89.

111. J. Cotter, K. Granger, R. Backx, et al. Social cognitive dysfunction as a clinical marker: a systematic review of meta-analyses across 30 clinical conditions. *Neurosci Biobehav Rev* 2018;**84**:92–9.

112. A.E. Richard, I.E. Scheffer, S.J. Wilson. Features of the broader autism phenotype in people with epilepsy support shared mechanisms between epilepsy and autism spectrum disorder. *Neurosci Biobehav Rev* 2018;**75**:203–33.

113. A.M. Kanner, J.J. Barry, F. Gilliam, et al. Anxiety disorders, subsyndromic depressive episodes, and major depressive episodes: do they differ on their impact on the quality of life of patients with epilepsy? *Epilepsia* 2010;**51**:1152–8.

114. G. Rayner, G.D. Jackson, SJ. Wilson. Two distinct symptom-based phenotypes of depression in epilepsy yield specific clinical and etiological insights. *Epilepsy Behav* 2016;**64**:336–44.

115. S. Paradiso, B.P. Hermann, D.P. Blumer, et al. Impact of depressed mood on neuropsychological status in temporal lobe epilepsy. *J Neurol Neurosurg Psychiatry* 2001;**70**:180–5.

116. J. Rösche, G. Kundt, R. Weber, et al. Memory deficits and depression in patients with chronic epilepsy. *Acta Neuropsychiatr* 2012;**24**:230–5.

117. C. Helmstaedter, M. Sonntag-Dillender, C. Hoppe, et al. Depressed mood and memory impairment in temporal lobe epilepsy as a function lateralization and localization. *Epilepsy Behav* 2004;**5**:696–701.

118. M.F. Dulay, B.K. Schefft, J.D. Fargo, et al. Severity of depressive symptoms, hippocampal sclerosis, auditory memory, and side of seizure focus in temporal lobe epilepsy. *Epilepsy Behav* 2004;**5**:522–31.

119. R.M. Busch, M.F. Dulay, K.H. Kim KH, et al. Pre-surgical mood predicts memory decline after anterior temporal lobe resection for epilepsy. *Arch Clin Neuropsychol* 2011;**26**:739–45.

120. M.F. Dulay, R.M. Busch, J.S. Chapin, et al. Executive functioning and depressed mood before and after unilateral frontal lobe resection for intractable epilepsy. *Neuropsychologia* 2013;**51**:1370–6.

121. S. Wiebe, W.T. Blume, J.P. Girvin, et al. Randomized, controlled trial of surgery for temporal-lobe epilepsy. *N Engl J Med* 2001;**345**:311–18.

122. S. Baxendale and P. Thompson. Red flags in epilepsy surgery: Identifying the patients who pay a high cognitive price for an unsuccessful surgical outcome. *Epilepsy Behav* 2018;**78**:269–72.

123. C. Helmstaedter, C.E. Elger, V.L. Vogt. Cognitive outcomes more than 5 years after temporal lobe epilepsy surgery: Remarkable functional recovery when seizures are controlled. *Seizure* 2018;**62**:116–23.

124. T. Gualtieri and D.R. Cox. The delayed neurobehavioural sequelae of traumatic brain injury. *Brain Inj* 1991;**5**:219–32.

125. L. Mazzini, F.M. Cossa, E. Angelino E, et al. Posttraumatic epilepsy: neuroradiologic and neuropsychological assessment of long-term outcome. *Epilepsia* 2003;**44**:569–74.

126. S. Dikmen and R.M. Reitan. Neuropsychological performance in posttraumatic epilepsy. *Epilepsia* 1978;**19**:177–83.

127. A.M. Haltiner, N.R. Temkin, H.R. Winn, et al. The impact of posttraumatic seizures on 1-year neuropsychological and psychosocial outcome of head injury. *J Int Neuropsychol Soc* 1996;**2**:494–504.

128. V. Raymont, A.M. Salazar, R. Lipsky, et al. Correlates of posttraumatic epilepsy 35 years following combat brain injury. *Neurology* 2010;**75**:224–9.

129. E. Farina, A. Raglio, A.R. Giovagnoli. Cognitive rehabilitation in epilepsy: An evidence-based review. *Epilepsy Res* 2015;**109**:210–18.

130. J.K. Kumar. Neuropsychological rehabilitation in neurological conditions: A circuitry approach. In: Kumar, J. K. (ed.) *Neuropsychological Rehabilitation: Principles and Applications.* 2012:103–22.

131. B.A. Wilson. Neuropsychological rehabilitation. *Annu Rev Clin Psychol* 2008;**4**:141–62.

132. M. Ylvisaker and T.J. Feeney *Collaborative Brain Injury Intervention: Positive Everyday Routines.* San Diego: Singular Publishing Group, 1998.

133. K. Postal and K. Armstrong. *Feedback that Sticks: The Art of Effectively Communicating Neuropsychological Assessment Results.* Oxford: Oxford University Press, 2013.

134. K.D. Cicerone, Y. Goldin, K. Ganci, *et al.* Evidence-based cognitive rehabilitation: systematic review of the literature from 2009 through 2014. *Arch Phys Med Rehabil* 2019;**100**:1515–33.

135. J. Ponsford, M. Bayley, C. Wiseman-Hakes, *et al.* INCOG recommendations for management of cognition following traumatic brain injury, part II: attention and information processing speed. *J Head Trauma Rehabil* 2014;**29**:321–37.

136. L. Fasotti, F. Kovacs, P.A.T.M. Eling, W. H. Brouwer. Time pressure management as a compensatory strategy training after closed head injury. *Neuropsychol Rehabil* 2000;**10**:47–65.

137. S. Sloan and J. Ponsford. Managing cognitive problems. In: Ponsford J.L., Sloan S., Snow P, eds. *Traumatic Brain Injury: Rehabilitation for Everyday Adaptive Living.* 2nd ed. London: Psychology Press, 2012;99–132.

138. M. Bayley, R. Teasell, S. Marshall S, *et al.* ABIKUS Evidence Based Recommendations for Rehabilitation of Moderate to Severe Acquired Brain Injury. Toronto, Ontario, Canada, Ontario Neurotrauma Foundation, 2007.

139. T.M. O'Neil-Pirozzi, M.R. Kennedy, M. M. Sohlberg. Evidence-based practice for the use of internal strategies as a memory compensation technique after brain injury: A systematic review. *J Head Trauma Rehabil* 2016;**31**:E1–1.

140. T.M. O'Neil-Pirozzi, G.E. Strangman, R. Goldstein, *et al.* A controlled treatment study of internal memory strategies (I-MEMS) following traumatic brain injury. *J Head Trauma Rehabil* 2010;**25**:43–51.

141. D. Velikonja, R. Tate, J. Ponsford, *et al.* INCOG recommendations for management of cognition following traumatic brain injury, part V: memory. *J Head Trauma Rehabil* 2010;**29**:369–86.

142. B.A. Wilson. *Memory Rehabilitation: Integrating Theory and Practice.* New York, NY: Guilford Press, 2009.

143. R. Tate, M. Kennedy, J. Ponsford, *et al.* INCOG recommendations for management of cognition following traumatic brain injury, part III: executive functioning and self-awareness. *J Head Trauma Rehabil* 2014;**29**:338–52.

144. M.R. Kennedy, C. Coelho, L. Turkstra, *et al.* Intervention for executive functions after traumatic brain injury: A systematic review, meta-analysis and clinical recommendations. *Neuropsychological Rehabil* 2008;**18**:257–99.

145. C. van Heugten, G. Wolters Gregório, D. Wade . Evidence-based cognitive rehabilitation after acquired brain injury: a systematic review of content of treatment. *Neuropsychological Rehabil* 2012;**22**:653–73.

146. P. Zoccolotti, A. Cantagallo, M. De Luca M, *et al.* Selective and integrated rehabilitation programs for disturbances of visual/spatial attention and executive function after brain damage: a neuropsychological evidence-based review. *Eur J Phys Rehabil Med* 2011;**47**:123–47.

147. J.M. Spikman, D.H.E. Boelen, K. F. Lamberts, *et al.* Effects of a multifaceted treatment program for executive dysfunction after acquired brain injury on indications of executive functioning in daily life. *J Int Neuropsychol Soc* 2010;**16**:118–29.

148. Y. Goverover, M.V. Johnston, J. Toglia, *et al.* Treatment to improve self-awareness in persons with acquired brain injury. *Brain Inj* 2007;**21**:913–23.

149. T. Ownsworth, J. Fleming, D. Shum, *et al.* Comparison of individual, group and combined intervention formats in

a randomized controlled trial for facilitating goal attainment and improving psychosocial function following acquired brain injury. *J Rehabil Med* 2008;**40**:81–8.

150. J. Schmidt, J. Fleming, T. Ownsworth, *et al*. Video feedback on functional task performance improves self-awareness after traumatic brain injury: a randomized controlled trial. *Neurorehabil Neural Repair* 2013;**27**:316–24.

151. A.K. Vas, S.B. Chapman, L.G. Cook, *et al*. Higher order reasoning training years after traumatic brain injury in adults. *J Head Trauma Rehabil* 2011;**26**:224–39.

152. C. Vallat-Azouvi, P. Azouvi, G. Le-Bornec, *et al*. Treatment of social cognition impairments in patients with traumatic brain injury: a critical review. *Brain Inj* 2019;**33**: 87–93.

153. C. Bornhofen and S. McDonald. Treating deficits in emotion perception following traumatic brain injury. *Neuropsychological Rehabil* 2008;**18**;22–44.

154. J.M. Guercio, H. Podolska-Schroeder, R. A. Rehfeldt. Using stimulus equivalence technology to teach emotion recognition to adults with acquired brain injury. *Brain Inj* 2004;**18**:593–601.

155. D. Neumann, D.R. Babbage, B. Zupan, *et al*. A randomized controlled trial of emotion recognition training after traumatic brain injury. *J Head Trauma Rehabil* 2015;**30**:E12–23.

156. J. Williamson and E. Isaki. Facial affect recognition training through telepractice: two case studies of individuals with chronic traumatic brain injury. *Int J Telerehabilitation* 2015;**7**:13–20.

157. J. Winegardner, C. Keohane, L. Prince, *et al*. Perspective training to treat anger problems after brain injury: two case studies. *NeuroRehabilitation* 2016;**39**:153–62.

158. T. Aboulafia-Brakha and R. Ptak. Effects of group psychotherapy on anger management following acquired brain injury. *Brain Inj* 2016;**30**:1121–30.

159. S. McDonald, R. Tate, L. Togher, *et al*. Social skills treatment for people with severe, chronic acquired brain injuries: a multicenter trial. *Arch Phys Med Rehabil* 2008;**89**:1648–59.

160. H.J. Westerhof-Evers, A.C. Visser-Keizer, L. Fasotti, *et al*. Effectiveness of a treatment for impairments in social cognition and emotion regulation (TScEmo) after traumatic brain injury: a randomized controlled trial. *J Head Trauma Rehabil* 2017;**32**:296–307.

161. A. Cassel, S. McDonald, M. Kelly, *et al*. Learning from the minds of others: A review of social cognition treatments and their relevance to traumatic brain injury. *Neuropsychological Rehabil* 2016;**29**:22–55.

162. S. Liu, X. Han, Y. Yan, *et al*. Quality of life and its influencing factors in patients with post-traumatic epilepsy. *Chin J Traumatol* 2011;**14**:100–3.

163. S.A. Kolakowsky-Hayner, J. Wright, J. Englander, *et al*. Impact of late post-traumatic seizures on physical health and functioning for individuals with brain injury within the community. *Brain Inj* 2013;**27**:578–86

164. P. Cuijpers, I.A. Cristea, E. Karyotaki, *et al*. How effective are cognitive behavior therapies for major depression and anxiety disorders? A meta-analytic update of the evidence. *World Psychiatry* 2016;**15**:245–58.

165. D.F. Tolin. Is cognitive-bhevaioural therapy more effective than other therapies? A meta-analytic review. *Clin Psychol Rev* 2010;**30**:710–20.

166. J. Ponsford, N. Lee, D. Wong, *et al*. Efficacy of motivational interviewing and cognitive behavioral therapy for anxiety and depression symptoms following traumatic brain injury. *Psychol Med* 2016;**46**:1079–90.

167. M. Gallagher, H.J. McLeod, T. M. McMillan. A systematic review of recommended modifications of CBT for people with cognitive impairments following brain injury. *Neuropsychological Rehabil* 2019;**29**:1–21.

168. T. Ownsworth and F. Gracey. Cognitive behavioural therapy for people with brain injury. In: Wilson, B. A. , Winegardner, J., van Heugten, C. M., Ownsworth, T. eds. *Neuropsychological Rehabilitation: The International Handbook*. Abingdon: Routledge, 2017;313–26

169. E. Grauwmeijer, M.H. Heijenbrok-Kal, I. K. Haitsma, *et al*. A prospective study on employment outcome 3 years after moderate to severe traumatic brain injury. *Arch Phys Med Rehabil* 2012;**93**:993–99.

170. R.R. Das and R.N. Moorthi. Traumatic brain injury in the war zone. *N Engl J Med* 2005;**353**:633–4.

171. V. Rao and C. Lyketsos. Neuropsychiatric sequelae of traumatic brain injury. *Psychosomatics* 2000;**41**:95–103.

172. M. Ono, T. Ownsworth, B. Walters. Preliminary investigation of misconceptions and expectations of the effects of traumatic brain injury and symptom reporting. *Brain Inj* 2011;**25**:237–49.

173. R.C.G. Chapman and J.M. Hudson. Beliefs about brain injury in Britain. *Brain Inj* 2010;**24**:797–801.

174. T.L. Swift and S.L. Wilson. Misconceptions about brain injury among the general public and non-expert health professionals: an exploratory study. *Brain Inj* 2001;**15**:149–65.

175. J. McClure, M.E. Devlin, J. McDowall, *et al*. Visible markers of brain injury influence attributions for adolescents' behaviour. *Brain Inj* 2006;**20**:1029–1035.

176. J. McClure. The role of causal attributions in public misconceptions about brain injury. *Rehabil Psychol* 2011;**56**:85–93.

177. J. Yu, H.M. Tam, T. Lee. Traumatic brain injury rehabilitation in Hong Kong: A review of practice and research. *Behav Neurol* 2015:274326.

178. M. Fresson, B. Dardenne, M. Geurten, *et al*. Stereotype content of people with acquired brain injury: Warm but incompetent. *J Appl Soc Psychol* 2017;**47**:539–52.

179. S. Koskinen, S. Quality of life 10 years after a very severe traumatic brain injury (TBI): The perspective of the injured and the closest relative. *Brain Inj* 1998;**12**:631–48.

180. E.J. Hicks, B.M. Larkins, S.C. Purdy. Fatigue management by speech-language pathologists for adults with traumatic brain injury. *Int J Speech Lang Pathol* 2011;**13**:145–55.

181. B. Johansson, P. Berglund, L. Ronnback. Mindfulness- based stress reduction (MBSR) improves long-term mental fatigue after stroke or traumatic brain injury. *Brain Inj* 2012;**26**: 1621–8.

182. S. Nguyen, A. McKay, D. Wong D, *et al*. Cognitive behavior therapy to treat sleep disturbance and fatigue after traumatic brain injury: A pilot randomized controlled trial. *Arch Phys Med Rehabil* 2017;**98**:1508–17.e2.

183. M. Daras, P. Bladin, M. Eadie, *et al*. Epilepsy: Historical perspectives. In. Engel J., Pedley T. A., Aicardi J., eds. *Epilepsy: a Comprehensive Textbook*. Philadelphia: Lippincott Williams & Wilkins, 2008.

184. G. Scrambler. Epilepsy, stigma and quality of life. *Neurol Asia* 2011;**16**:35–6.

185. A. Jacoby, G.A. Baker, N. Steen, *et al*. The clinical course of epilepsy and its psychosocial correlates: findings from a U.K. community study. *Epilepsia* 1996;**37**:148–61.

186. M. Bishop, C.A. Allen. The impact of epilepsy on quality of life: a qualitative analysis. *Epilepsy Behav* 2003;**4**: 226–33.

Chapter

Neuropsychiatric Consequences of Moderate to Severe Traumatic Brain Injury

Niruj Agrawal

Introduction

Neuropsychiatric consequences of moderate to severe traumatic brain injury (TBI) include various emotional and neurobehavioural problems such as mood swings, impulsivity, apathy, irritability, agitation, aggression, depression, anxiety and psychosis. Using Schedule for Clinical Assessment in Neuropsychiatry (SCAN) interviews, Deb et al. found that at 1 year from a TBI, there were more people with an ICD10 diagnosis of a psychiatric condition as than in the general population.[1] However, rates for psychiatric symptoms that did not fulfil diagnostic criteria for a specific psychiatric condition as per formal diagnostic criteria were much higher. This finding is consistent with the clinical experience with post-TBI cases where neuropsychiatric presentation are often more varied, atypical and may not meet the diagnostic threshold for common psychiatric conditions.

In a 30-year follow-up study, using DSM-IV criteria, a 48.3% prevalence of Axis I disorders and 23.3% for Axis II personality disorders were reported that started after TBI.[2] The most common psychiatric diagnoses following TBI included major depression (26.7%), alcohol abuse or dependence (11.7%), panic disorder (8.3%), specific phobia (8.3%) and psychotic disorders (6.7%). People with TBI were nearly twice more likely to have psychiatric problems than general population.

A prospective 5-year study reported a 75.2% prevalence of Axis I disorders according to DSM-IV criteria, the large majority of these conditions (77.7%) starting during the first year after the TBI.[3] Anxiety, mood and substance-use disorders were the most common diagnostic classes, often presenting co-morbidly. The strongest predictors of post-TBI psychiatric disorders were pre-injury disorder and accident-related limb injury.

Figure 9.1 schematically represents a range of common neuropsychiatric problems seen after moderate to severe TBI. These conditions will be discussed in greater detail in the subsequent sections.

Mood Disorders

Mood disorders are a common consequence of TBI and include depression and other persistent milder mood disorders such as dysthymia. Depression, in particular, is associated with subjective distress, poor outcomes, increased dysfunction and has the potential to affect quality of life significantly.

Fann et al reported depression in up to 60% of patients with TBI in the first year after TBI but prevalence rates range from 17% to 60% depending on screening tools, study populations, study design and diagnostic criteria/threshold used which determines the variability in the prevalence rates.[4] People who had a pre TBI depression or ongoing

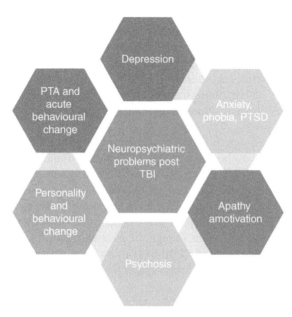

Figure 9.1 Neuropsychiatric problems following traumatic brain injury.

depression at the time of TBI are more likely to have more significant and persistent depression post-TBI.[5]

Depression following TBI can be caused by a number of factors including biological, psychological and social factors which often overlap.[6] Psychological factors comprise reaction to psychological trauma, loss of function, loss of role, diminished tolerance to frustration, low self-esteem and maladaptive coping strategies. Social factors encompass lack of adequate social support, difficulties with relationships, unrealistic expectations and involvement in litigation. Biological factors include brain lesions in the frontal and temporal lobes disrupting neural networks between the prefrontal cortex, amygdala, hippocampus, basal ganglia and thalamus, neurochemical and neuroendocrinal abnormalities, such as serotonergic deficits and hypothalamic–pituitary–adrenal axis function are frequently associated with depression after TBI.[7] These biological, psychological and social factors commonly co-exist and interact with each other and good clinical assessment should take into account all of these factors.

Major depressive disorder after TBI is often associated with poorer cognitive functioning, aggression and anxiety, greater functional disability, poorer recovery and greater health care costs.[5] Depression is also an independent predictor of poorer health-related quality of life after TBI. People who sustained a TBI with structural brain lesions have a four times increased risk of suicide as compared to the general population.[8] A retrospective study on veterans showed that suicide risk is associated with depression, partner relationship problems and family circumstance problems, but not with TBI severity, alcohol dependence or post-traumatic stress disorder (PTSD). However, odds for suicide seem to increase with the number of psychiatric comorbidities with three psychiatric comorbidities being associated with 6.5 times increased risk of suicide, highlighting the importance of identifying and treating psychiatric conditions associated with TBI.[9]

In terms of differential diagnosis, it is important to bear in mind that a number of symptoms of depression could overlap with core features of TBI including tiredness, poor concentration, sleep and appetite changes. This makes the assessment of depression more difficult. Depression should ideally be routinely screened either though use of standardised depression screening instruments followed by full neuropsychiatric assessment. Attempts should be made to rule out conditions that could lead on to symptoms similar to depressive symptoms after TBI. These include conditions such as hypopituitarism and apathy-amotivation.

Affective dysregulation due to frontal lobe damage may also be confused with depression. There may be sudden outbursts of crying or laughter, without any obvious reason that even surprise the patient. This is often called pathological laughter/crying or called pseudobulbar affect. This is different from the emotional lability associated with frontal lobe dysfunction, where there are constant changes in emotions. These cases can be misdiagnosed as depression if the crying spells are frequent, but this should be avoided for diagnostic clarity and prognosis, even though the pharmacological treatment is similar to depression. These cases benefit from use of SSRI medication with evidence being best for citalopram. Psychological approaches such as cognitive behavioural therapy (CBT) are not helpful for this condition.

In terms of treatment, antidepressants are considered to be effective in treating depression in neurological settings.[10] Clinicians should have a low threshold for diagnosing and treating depression post-TBI given the costs for not doing so in terms of outcomes and quality of life. A systematic review looking at treatment for depression after TBI showed that SSRIs and cognitive behavioural interventions appear to have the best preliminary evidence for treating depression following TBI.[4] Sertraline and citalopram seem to be well tolerated. Clinically, as a routine these are recommended as a first line treatment for post-TBI depression. Tricyclic antidepressants do not have good evidence for efficacy and have a higher risk of side effects and are generally avoided. Monoamine oxidase inhibitors (MAOIs) are not recommended due to a lack of efficacy data and potentially serious side effects, specifically with difficulties in adhering to dietary restrictions due to cognitive difficulties. Psychological treatments such as CBT have comparable efficacy to antidepressants and are first line approach for milder symptoms or combined with pharmacological treatment for moderate to severe depression. Other psychological treatments often used include goal setting, behavioural activation and problem solving therapy in multidisciplinary neurorehabilitation settings.[11]

Anxiety Disorders

A wide spectrum of anxiety disorders can develop following a TBI, including acute stress reaction, generalised anxiety disorder (GAD), specific phobic anxiety, social phobia, panic disorders, obsessive compulsive disorder (OCD) or post-traumatic stress disorder (PTSD). Some of these anxiety disorders such as acute stress reaction are transient and settle with time. Others such as phobic anxiety can be persistent and distressing and may affect an individual's functioning quite significantly. While travel-related anxiety is fairly common after road traffic accidents, other specific phobias could relate to stairs after a fall and going out to public places in cases of assaults. These can be highly disabling with a huge impact on functioning and in some cases on finances.

A large prospective cohort study on post-TBI anxiety showed a high proportion of participants suffered from significant levels of anxiety during the first year post-TBI regardless of TBI severity and gender. At 4, 8 and 12 months, respectively, 29.9%, 29.2% and 30.8% of participants presented clinically significant anxiety symptoms.[12] Participants with a positive premorbid history of anxiety disorders had greater anxiety on the Hospital Anxiety and Depression Scale (HADS) compared to those with a negative premorbid anxiety history. Prevalence rates for various anxiety disorder following TBI is reported based on kind of anxiety disorder including panic disorder 8.3%, specific phobia of 8.3% and generalised anxiety disorder of 1.7%.[2]

Patients with TBI can also experience other physical and psychological symptoms of trauma including fear of death or fear of subsequent treatment.[13] These traumatic experiences may result in or contribute to the development of PTSD. The diagnosis of PTSD may be difficult following TBI because of overlap with symptoms of TBI particularly with post-concussion syndrome. In addition, various behavioural symptoms following the TBI such as increased alcohol consumption, depression, impulsivity or irritability may also alter PTSD presentation making it harder to diagnose. However, PTSD rates after a TBI are approximately five times higher than those reported in the general population.[14, 15] Rates of PTSD are higher in mild TBI than severe TBI. Disruption to memory and cognitive function in severe TBI are considered to be a protective factor. However, there have been reports that PTSD can occur after TBI even when there is a significant disturbance of consciousness or disrupted memory for the trauma.[14]

PTSD presents with symptoms of intrusive memories such as flashbacks and nightmares, avoidance of reminders of the trauma and hyperarousal. PTSD is commonly associated with co-morbid psychiatric conditions. Most common of these are depression, substance misuse and other anxiety disorders. People suffering from co-morbid PTSD and TBI complain of more severe neurocognitive symptoms and disability. Sleep disturbance is common in PTSD after TBI and may hinder recovery if not treated. PTSD commonly affects behaviour and may exacerbate TBI-associated irritability, agitation and aggression. The relationship between PTSD, TBI and epilepsy is discussed in Chapter 11.

Diagnosis of anxiety disorders following a TBI requires careful consideration of the overlap between anxiety disorders, depression and other neurobehavioral disorders due to TBI. Treatment of anxiety is best managed as part of neurorehabilitation care at a multidisciplinary level with a combination of anxiety management techniques, CBT and pharmacological treatments with SSRI.

Apathy

Apathy or amotivation is not uncommon following TBI and can be misdiagnosed as depression. Apathy has been described using a variety of terms including amotivation and abulia but it is not simply a lack of motivation as it is associated with reduced goal-directed behaviour, impaired initiative, diminished activity and lack of concern. Furthermore, a distinction should be made between apathy as a symptom of mood disorder, altered level of consciousness or cognitive impairment and apathy as a syndrome of acquired changes in mood, behaviour and cognition, not due to mood disorder, altered level of consciousness or cognitive impairment.[16] Symptoms of apathy are commonly divided into three dimensions: behavioural, cognitive and emotional. Assessment consists of a good history and account of symptoms from carers and wider multidisciplinary team, measures such as the Apathy Evaluation Scale can help with diagnosis.[17]

Apathy is associated with poor outcomes due to lack of engagement in neurorehabilitation and may impact on family, social and occupational functioning of patients and can cause increased caregiver distress.

Treatment of mild cases can be based on cognitive interventions while more severe cases require a combination of pharmacological and non-pharmacological approaches. Cognitive interventions are the most commonly used strategy but other interventions such as music therapy and cognitive rehabilitation have also been used.[18] Behavioural approaches such as activity scheduling are also used. Pharmacological treatments include dopaminergic drugs such as selegiline, stimulants such as methylphenidate and modafinil, cholinesterase inhibitors such as donepezil and SSRIs.

Psychosis

While some consider post-TBI psychosis controversial, accumulating evidence is pointing towards a higher prevalence (up to 7 times) of psychosis following TBI as compared to general population. Rates of psychosis in TBI are estimated to be up to 10% but ranging between 1.35% and 9.2%.[19] Risk factors include male gender, alcohol and substance use, including cannabis and pre-existing psychiatric conditions like depression. Frontal, temporal or hippocampal lesions, as well as memory dysfunction and impairment of executive functions, seem also to be associated. The development of post-traumatic epilepsy (PTE) or subclinical epileptiform discharges can also be a contributory factor.

Psychosis following TBI most commonly presents as a delusional disorder or a schizophrenia-like psychosis. Delusional disorders may present with specific syndromes such as Capgras' syndrome, reduplicative paramnesia, delusional jealousy, Cotard's syndrome or somatic delusions (11%). Schizophrenia-like psychosis commonly presents with auditory hallucinations, persecutory delusions and negative symptoms. The onset of a psychosis after TBI could be delayed by years with a mean latency ranging between 3 and 5 years while delusional disorders tend to develop in the first year after TBI.[20]

Clinical assessment should focus on establishing the phenomenology of psychotic symptoms and rule out other causes including substance induced psychosis, epilepsy-related psychosis and a primary psychotic disorder. Initial post-TBI presentation with agitation and behavioural problems associated with post-traumatic amnesia can be confused with psychosis. Diagnosis of psychosis should be avoided when the patient is still in post-traumatic amnesia. Treatment of psychosis after TBI is not different from the treatment of any other psychotic disorder but special consideration should be given to interactions with other medication, sensitivity to side effects and impact on neurocognitive functions.

Acute Behavioural Changes and Post-Traumatic Amnesia

Post-traumatic amnesia (PTA) can last from minutes to months depending on the severity of TBI and is commonly associated with agitation, disruptive behaviour, impulsivity and aggression. In the initial aftermath of TBI, there is commonly a transient state of inability to encode new memories, difficulty sustaining attention associated with confusion and disorientation along with lack of insight and awareness.[21] This state is called PTA. Duration of PTA is commonly used as a reliable measure of severity of TBI along with other indices such as Glasgow Coma Scale (GCS) score and duration of loss of consciousness. It is now widely recognised that PTA is an important predictor of functional outcome after a TBI.

In addition to cognitive and behavioural difficulties including agitation, PTA is commonly associated with disordered language and cognitive communication impairments. Confusion may also manifest in communication impairments such as confabulation, perseveration and disorganised discourse[22] as well as autonomic changes associated in form of tachycardia, transient pyrexia and clamminess.[21] PTA can be associated with focal lesions and decreased cerebral perfusion in the frontal and temporal lobes.[23]

However, agitation can be due to a number of other causes including epilepsy, particularly non-convulsive status, depression, frontal lobe and paralimbic pathology as well as withdrawal states. There is no clear association with gender or age. Post-TBI agitation can be associated with higher chances of subsequent neuropsychiatric problems. Worse outcome for agitation are associated with a longer duration of agitation, severity of agitation behaviour and structural abnormalities on brain scan.[24]

Assessment of PTA include scales such as the Westmead PTA Scale[25] but a detailed assessment of agitated patient after TBI will not only involve assessment of PTA but will require a detailed neuropsychiatric assessment to establish past and family history of psychiatric problems including any personality issues, alcohol and substance misuse and doing a detailed mental state examination. This helps establish the cause of agitation and clarify if there are any other co-morbid psychiatric conditions present.

Management of agitated behaviour during the PTA requires careful management of environment with minimisation of excessive stimulation, reorientation and avoidance of restraints while maintain safety. A wide range of pharmacological agents has been used in agitation following TBI but evidence for any pharmacological agent or even drug class is poor. Currently no medication is approved for treatment of agitation after TBI. Nevertheless, various medications, including beta blockers, atypical antipsychotics (e.g. risperidone) and antiepileptic agents (e.g. carbamazepine and valproate), are widely used in the management of patients with acute agitation or aggression. However, a Cochrane review showed that only high doses of beta blockers seem to be effective in controlling agitation following TBI but the two controls trials included in this review involved a small number of patients and this finding has not been replicated.[26] This review did not find enough evidence for efficacy of other agents such as valproate or carbamazepine. Use of beta blockers needs to be carefully monitored due to its effect on blood pressure and chances of inducing falls due to postural hypotension. A recent French guideline noted that there are no standards or consensus regarding the use of neuroleptics. Greater sensitivity to their adverse effects post-TBI was noted.[27]

The antiepileptic agents carbamazepine (CBZ) and valproate (VPA) are commonly used as mood stabilisers to treat agitation after TBI. The North American neurobehavioral guideline working group noted that carbamazepine seems to be effective for some patients experiencing aggression after TBI, though the published literature did not support a recommendation for use of carbamazepine at that time.[28] They concluded that there is insufficient evidence to support the development of any standards for the treatment of aggression following TBI. More recently, a French guideline noted that carbamazepine and valproate were effective for treatment of agitation and aggression and are recommended as first line treatment.[27] Other antiepileptic agents such as oxcarbazepine, lamotrigine and gabapentin do not have any evidence to support their use. Levetiracetam has no positive effect on aggressiveness post-TBI and can make agitation and aggressiveness worse along with the risks of behavioural and mood disorders, hence should be avoided.

Benzodiazepines can sometimes be used in acute emergency for sedation, but generally their regular use should be avoided as they can have negative effects on neurocognition and can make aggression paradoxically worse. Other pharmacological agents which have been tried for agitation and aggression following TBI include amantadine, buspirone, modafinil and methylphenidate. Out of these agents methylphenidate seems to be most promising though further evidence is required before routine clinical use can be recommended.

Long-term Personality and Behavioural Changes

TBI is associated with a number of behavioural and personality changes including impulsivity, disinhibition and aggression along with emotional dyscontrol. They are generally pervasive, prolonged and causes distress and/or dysfunction to reach the clinical threshold of diagnosis. Manifestations of personality change commonly overlap with changes in mood, sleep, fatigue and cognitive functions. These personality and behavioural changes can be significant barriers to engagement in neurorehabilitation and can have a negative impact on recovery and ability to return back to work. It is noted that patients with organic personality disorder (OPD) after TBI develop more psychosocial adjustment and emotional problems than patients with TBI without OPD diagnosis. This difference is independent of severity of cognitive impairments or severity of injury based on GCS score.[29]

Hibbard et al reported around 66% of personality disorder in a group of patients with TBI but no correlation with TBI severity, age at injury and time since injury.[30] A 30-year follow-up study, reported at least one personality disorder in about 23.3%.[2] Other authors have suggested severity of brain injury measured as duration of loss of consciousness and degree of cognitive impairment as an important predictor of personality changes following TBI.[31]

Personality changes are associated with poor psychosocial adjustment, poor emotional functioning, increased care giver distress, poor engagement with rehabilitative treatment and poor occupational functioning. Frontal lobe lesions (particularly orbitofrontal area), anterior temporal lesions, disruption to limbic system and impairment of frontal lobe functions on neurocognitive assessment are commonly associated with organic personality change. Widespread damage caused by shearing stress such as diffuse axonal injury can commonly result in organic personality change. However, personality changes can occur in absence of any discernible cognitive impairment or without any identifiable structural brain lesions. Individuals with pre-existing psychiatric conditions or personality disorders can be at a greater risk of developing organic personality change. In absence of structural lesion patients may present with a combination of exacerbation of pre-existing personality traits, organic orderliness and obsessionality, adjustment to post injury life along with persistent irritability and morbid anxiety impacting on personality and behaviour.

Clinical assessment should include assessment of current and past axis I psychiatric conditions, assessment of neurocognitive functions and collateral history from family and carers. Detailed neurocognitive assessment helps in establishing nature and severity of neurocognitive difficulties which may have an impact on behaviour. Specific measures such as the Frontal Systems Behaviour Scale (FrSBe), Behaviour Rating Inventory of Executive Functions (BRIEF) and Dysexecutive Questionnaire (DEX questionnaire) can be used to help with diagnosis. Management of organic personality change is best delivered in the context of brain injury rehabilitative services with a combination of behavioural programme and pharmacological management. Currently the evidence base to support the pharmacological treatment remain poor but agents such as selective serotonin reuptake inhibitors (SSRIs), mood stabilisers such as carbamazepine and atypical antipsychotic agents such as risperidone are commonly used in clinical practice. Other agents tried include stimulants such as methylphenidate and dopaminergic drugs such as bromocriptine. These are more likely to be used when there is an overlap with apathy symptoms.

Considerations for Alcohol and Drug Use

Alcohol and drug use is a common problem in people with TBI before and after TBI. Alcohol is considered to be a major risk factor for injury with 30% to 50% patients intoxicated at the time of a brain injury.[32] Alcohol consumption on the day of injury is well recognised to increase the risk of sustaining a TBI, but the evidence so far suggests that alcohol consumption on the day of injury does not appear to be associated with substantially poorer outcomes after TBI.[33] However, alcohol use after TBI carries several risks. These include increased risk of recurrent TBI, more atrophy of the cerebral cortex, development of PTE and deterioration of behavioural functioning.[34] In addition people may have worsening of neurocognitive difficulties, increased emotional difficulties and aggression.

Substance abuse is also a risk factor for TBI due to impact on cognitive function, behaviour and judgment. Substance misuse pre and post-TBI is commonly associated with alcohol misuse. Approximately 50% to 60% of persons with TBI have significant issues with alcohol and/or drugs.[35] A history of substance abuse predicts increased disability, worse symptomatology, poorer prognosis and delayed recovery. Substance misuse post injury could lead on to problems with emotions, behaviour, motivation, neurocognitive functions and overall outcome from TBI.

Special Considerations for Post-traumatic Epilepsy

Both epilepsy and TBI are associated with a wide range of psychiatric problems. Hence it is probable that PTE in the aftermath of TBI should present with comorbid psychiatric symptoms. So far, the evidence points to an increased risk of psychiatric problems in patients with TBI who develop PTE as compared to those who do not.[36] However, this still remains a relatively unexplored area with a number of questions remaining unanswered concerning the genetic and environmental contributors, the phenomenology of psychiatric disorders in PTE and how to prevent and treat them adequately.[37]

Whilst considering neuropsychiatric aspects of PTE, a number of factors have to be considered, including the severity of the TBI, the site of the brain lesion and the presence of cognitive problems along with any co-morbid alcohol and substance misuse.[37] All these factors can profoundly affect the phenomenology of any psychiatric condition. In addition, the potential effect of antiepileptic drugs could be an important factor in psychiatric symptomatology as in patients with epilepsy. People with a severe TBI may be more sensitive to neurocognitive, emotional and neurobehavioural side effects of antiepileptic drugs.

Patients with TBI who develop PTE are noted to be more likely to develop personality changes, like disinhibited and aggressive behaviours, as compared with those who did not.[36] These personality changes were noted to be unrelated to the development of neurocognitive problems.

Epidemiological evidence currently points to an association between the presence of depression at the time of the TBI, or as a consequence of it, with an increased risk of developing epilepsy.[38] However, there are no studies that specifically investigated the phenomenology of depression in PTE as compared with that of people with TBI without epilepsy or other epilepsy syndromes.[37]

TBI and epilepsy are known to be associated with risk of psychosis. However, no studies have investigated the prevalence of psychosis in PTE and the potential role of PTE in the development of a psychotic disorder. It is important to clarify in the future studies whether people with PTE are more likely to present with psychotic symptoms and whether they progress more rapidly from postictal psychoses to a chronic inter-ictal psychosis than patients with other epilepsy syndromes.[37]

The diagnosis and management of psychiatric disorders in PTE can be even more challenging than in other epilepsy syndromes due to the complexity of additional co-morbidities of TBI and lack of evidence on impact of PTE on phenomenology of neuro-psychiatric symptoms. In the future, it will be important to clarify whether prompt treatment of any psychiatric disorder after TBI can affect the chances of developing epilepsy, to explore drug classes which can potentially address psychiatric disorders and epilepsy at the same time and whether standard of care for psychiatric disorders outside PTE is equally effective in psychiatric comorbidities of PTE.[37]

Post-TBI in addition to increased risk of PTE, there can be increased risk of functional seizures. A study found increased incident of past brain injury in a cohort of people with functional seizures.[39] They concluded that head trauma may be a frequent precipitant to psychogenic non-epileptic seizures. The injury severity levels were predominantly mild or minimal (85%), which is in contrast to the relative risk of epilepsy after mild or minimal head injury and is widely accepted to be no greater than the risk for the general population. They concluded that mild head injury plays a substantially larger role as a risk factor in the epidemiology of functional seizures than it does in epilepsy. Similar results were reported by another group,[40] who found that 24% of people with functional seizures had the onset of their seizures attributed to a head injury. The majority (78%) of patients with functional seizures sustained only mild head injury. It was noted that patients with functional seizures after head injury resemble patients with persistent post-concussional syndrome with symptoms closely associated including poor concentration and memory, headache and other episodic neurologic symptoms.

Conclusions

Patients with TBI need to be managed within multidisciplinary trauma pathways with involvement of various therapists including neuropsychologists, physiotherapists, occupational therapists and speech and language therapists. Neuropsychiatrist should be an integral part of such teams. Treatments are individualised following detailed assessment of a patient's problems and their strengths and weaknesses using goal-planning approach. Neuropsychiatric conditions following TBI are treated in such a context with a combination of pharmacological, psychological, behavioural and social approaches. It is yet unclear whether development of PTE changes the phenomenology of neuropsychiatric presentation after TBI or the outcome to their treatment.

Pharmacological approaches require attention to issues specific to TBI including sensitivity to side effects, impact on energy levels and cognitive functions and interactions with other medications and PTE. Almost any psychotropic medication which is used for any psychiatric disorder has been used in patients following TBI. This is a growing field with gradual accumulation of evidence. Currently, no medications are specifically approved to be used post-TBI by FDA, European and UK regulators. General rule is to start low and go slow and remove medications, which are not helpful with regular planned reviews.

References

1. Deb, S., Lyons, I., Koutzoukis, C., Ali, I. and McCarthy, G. 1999. Rate of psychiatric illness 1 year after traumatic brain injury. *Am J Psychiatr* 156: 374–8.

2. Koponen, S., Taiminen, T., Portin, R., et al. 2002. Axis I and II psychiatric disorders after traumatic brain injury: a 30-year follow-up study. *Am J Psychiatr* 159:1315–21.

3. Alway, Y., Gould, K.R., Johnston, L., McKenzie, D. and Ponsford, J. 2016. A prospective examination of Axis I psychiatric disorders in the first 5 years following moderate to severe traumatic brain injury. *Psychol Med* 46:1331–41.

4. Fann, J.R., Hart, T. and Schomer, K.G. 2009. Treatment for depression after traumatic brain injury: a systematic review. *J Neurotrauma* 26:2383–402.

5. Bombardier, C.H., Fann, J.R., Temkin, N.R., Esselman, P.C., Barber, J. and Dikmen, S.S. 2010. Rates of major depressive disorder and clinical outcomes following traumatic brain injury. JAMA, 303:1938–45.

6. Osborn, A.J., Mathias, J.L. and Fairweather-Schmidt, A.K. 2014. Depression following adult, non-penetrating traumatic brain injury: A meta-analysis examining methodological variables and sample characteristics. *Neurosci Biobehav Rev* 47:1–15.

7. Jorge, R.E. and Starkstein. S.E. 2005. Pathophysiologic aspects of major depression following traumatic brain injury. *J Head Trauma Rehabil* 20:475–87.

8. Teasdale, T.W. and Engberg, A.W. 2001. Suicide after traumatic brain injury: a population study. *J Neurol Neurosurg Psychiatr* 71:436–40.

9. Skopp N.A., Trofimovich L., Grimes J., Oetjen-Gerdes L. and Gahm G.A. Relations between suicide and traumatic brain injury, psychiatric diagnoses, and relationship problems, active component, US Armed Forces, 2001–2009. Air Force Medical Support Agency Fort Detrick MD Air Force Medical Evaluation Support Activity; 2012 Feb.

10. Agrawal, N. and Rickards, H. 2011. Detection and treatment of depression in neurological disorders. *J Neurol Neurosurg Psychiatr* 82:828–9.

11. Cuijpers, P., van Straten, A. and Wamerdam, L. 2007. Problem solving therapies for depression: A meta-analysis. *Eur Psychiatry* 22:9–15.

12. Laviolette, V., Ouellet, M.C., Beaulieu-Bonneau, S. and Giguere, M. 2014. Anxiety in the first year after traumatic brain injury: Evolution and risk factors. *Brain Injury* 28:705–6.

13. Hiott, D.W. and Labbate, L. 2002. Anxiety disorders associated with traumatic brain injuries. *NeuroRehabilitation* 17:345–55.

14. Rogers, J.M. and Read, C.A. 2007. Psychiatric comorbidity following traumatic brain injury. *Brain Injury* 21:1321–33.

15. Tanev, K.S., Pentel, K.Z., Kredlow, M.A. and Charney, M.E. 2014. PTSD and TBI co-morbidity: scope, clinical presentation and treatment options. *Brain Injury* 28:261–70.

16. van Reekum, R., Stuss, D.T. and Ostrander, L. 2005. Apathy: why care? *J Neuropsychiatry and Clinical Neurosci* 17:7–19.

17. Marin, R.S., Biedrzycki, R.C. and Firinciogullar, S. 1991. Reliability and validity of the Apathy Evaluation Scale. *Psychiatry Res* 38:143–62.

18. Lane-Brown, A.T. and Tate, R.L. 2009. Apathy after acquired brain impairment: a systematic review of non-pharmacological interventions. *Neuropsychol Rehabil* 19:481–516.

19. Batty, R.A., Rossell. S.L., Francis. A.J. and Ponsford, J. 2013. Psychosis following traumatic brain injury. *Brain Impairment* 14:21–41.

20. Fujii, D.E. and Ahmed, I. 2014. Psychotic disorder caused by traumatic brain injury. *Psychiatr Clin North Am* 37:113–24.

21. Marshman, L.A., Jakabek, D., Hennessy, M., Quirk, F. and Guazzo, E.P. 2013. Post-traumatic amnesia. *J Clin Neurosci* 20:1475–81.

22. Steel, J., Ferguson, A., Spencer, E. and Togher, L. 2015. Language and cognitive communication during post-traumatic amnesia: A critical synthesis. *NeuroRehabilitation* 37:221–34.

23. Metting, Z., Rödiger, L.A., de Jong, B.M., Stewart, R.E., Kremer, B.P. and van der Naalt J. 2010. Acute cerebral perfusion CT abnormalities associated with posttraumatic amnesia in mild head injury. *J Neurotrauma* 27:2183–9.

24. Singh, R., Venkateshwara, G., Nair, K.P., Khan, M. and Saad, R. 2014. Agitation after traumatic brain injury and predictors of outcome. *Brain Injury* 28:336–40.

25. Shores, E.A., Marosszeky, J.E., Sandanam, J. and Batchelor, J. 1986. Preliminary validation of a scale for measuring the duration of post-traumatic amnesia. *Medical J Australia*, 144:569–72.

26. Fleminger, S., Greenwood, R.R. and Oliver, D.L. 2003. Pharmacological management for agitation and aggression in people with acquired brain injury. *Cochrane Database of Systematic Reviews*. 2006(4):CD003299.

27. Plantier, D. and Luauté, J. 2016. Drugs for behavior disorders after traumatic brain injury: systematic review and expert consensus leading to French recommendations for good practice. *Ann Phys Rehabil Med* 59:42–57.

28. Warden D.L., Gordon B, McAllister T.W., et al. 2006. Guidelines for the pharmacologic treatment of neurobehavioral sequelae of traumatic brain injury. *J Neurotrauma* 23:1468–501.

29. Franulic, A., Horta, E., Maturana, R., Scherpenisse, J. and Carbonell, C. 2000. Organic personality disorder after traumatic brain injury: Cognitive, anatomic and psychosocial factors. A 6 month follow-up. *Brain Injury* 14:431–9.

30. Hibbard, M.R., Bogdany, J., Uysal, S., et al. 2000. Axis II psychopathology in individuals with traumatic brain injury. *Brain Injury* 14:45–61.

31. Golden, Z. and Golden, C.J. 2003. Impact of brain injury severity on personality dysfunction. *Int J Neuroscience* 113:733–45.

32. Tien, H.C., Tremblay, L.N., Rizoli, S.B., et al. 2006. Association between alcohol and mortality in patients with severe traumatic head injury. *Arch Surg* 141:1185–91.

33. Mathias, J.L. and Osborn, A.J. 2018. Impact of day-of-injury alcohol consumption on outcomes after traumatic brain injury: A meta-analysis. *Neuropsychol Rehabil* 28:997–1018.

34. Opreanu, R.C., Kuhn, D. and Basson, M.D. 2010. Influence of alcohol on mortality in traumatic brain injury. *J Am Coll Surg* 210:997–1007.

35. Allen, S., Stewart, S.H., Cusimano, M. and Asbridge, M. 2016. Examining the relationship between traumatic brain injury and substance use outcomes in the Canadian population. *Subst Use Misuse* 51:1577–86.

36. Mazzini, L., Cossa, F.M., Angelino, E., Campini, R., Pastore, I. and Monaco F. 2003. Posttraumatic epilepsy: neuroradiologic and neuropsychological assessment of long-term outcome. *Epilepsia* 44:569–74.

37. Mula M. 2019. Psychiatric aspects of posttraumatic epilepsy: A still

unexplored area. *Epilepsy Behav* 101:106598.

38. Rapoport M.J., McCullagh S., Shammi P. and Feinstein A. 2005. Cognitive impairment associated with major depression following mild and moderate traumatic brain injury. *J Neuropsychiatry Clin Neurosci* 17:61–5

39. Westbrook, L.E., Devinsky, O. and Geocadin, R. 1998. Nonepileptic seizures after head injury. *Epilepsia* 39:978–82.

40. Barry E., Krumholz A., Bergey G.K., Chatha H., Alemayehu S. and Grattan L. 1998. Nonepileptic posttraumatic seizures. *Epilepsia* 39:427–31.

Chapter 10

Traumatic Brain Injury and Psychogenic Nonepileptic Seizures

David K. Chen and W. Curt LaFrance

Introduction

Psychogenic nonepileptic seizures (PNES) are paroxysms of altered sensory, cognitive and/or motor manifestations, with or without alteration in consciousness that may resemble epileptic seizures (ES), but do not originate from abnormal electrical brain activity. Most presentations of PNES fulfill criteria for Functional Neurological Symptom Disorder (Conversion Disorder – CD) under *Diagnostic and Statistical Manual of Mental Disorders, Fifth Edition* (DSM-5),[1] reflecting a seizure type in which psychological conflicts are converted to somatic ES-like symptoms. The classic psychological process is described as, when focusing on external seizure manifestations (or other somatic symptoms), the patient's own internal stressors (e.g., the weights of self-culpability surrounding psychological conflicts and/or self-responsibility to resolve them) are alleviated from conscious awareness. [2]

Several etiological frameworks exist for CD of seizure type. No single mechanism or contributing factor has been known to be necessary and sufficient to explain all heterogeneous cases of PNES or any other CD manifestation. [3] One framework conceives PNES as arising from a biopsychosocial, multifactorial etiologic model as illustrated in Figure 10.1. PNES are conceptualized to evolve from serial interacting factors over time, comprised of Predisposing, Precipitating and Perpetuating factors.[4, 5] *Predisposing* factors consist of inherent or imbued elements within the patient's constitution, which confer vulnerability

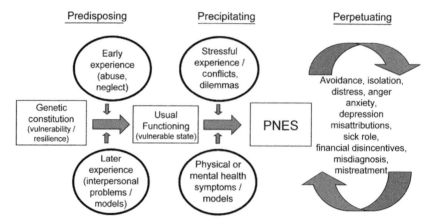

Figure 10.1 Biopsychosocial etiological model: Development of psychogenic nonepileptic seizures via multifactorial contributions including Predisposing, Precipitating and Perpetuating factors. From Reuber, with permission.[6]

toward eventual development of PNES later in life. *Precipitating* events occur in individual's lives which patients may identify as "the cause" (e.g., a head injury, an assault, a blast exposure). *Perpetuating* factors, both internal and external, aggravate the underlying conflicts/issues. Whereas one factor may appear to play predominant roles in a particular patient, this model stipulates that other important factors may also be involved and should not be overlooked.[6]

Studies have reported a notably high co-occurrence rate of PNES and traumatic brain injury (TBI), with a weighted average of 43% among 1,039 adult patients with PNES across 17 studies.[7] While PNES have an estimated prevalence of 2–33/100,000 (more in women)[8] and a history of TBI is endorsed by 12% of the general population in developed countries (mostly men),[9] it is unlikely that coincidental co-occurrence can entirely explain such high comorbidity of PNES and TBI. In applying the biopsychosocial model, this review discusses how TBI may subserve contributing roles as Predisposing, Precipitating and Perpetuating factors in the development of PNES.

Structural or Functional Effects of TBI as Predisposing/Precipitating Factors

Earlier investigations have shown that in cases where PNES were preceded by TBI, 87% of such cases occur with mild TBI (mTBI),[10] while 13–33% were with moderate to severe TBI.[10, 11] Both of these cited studies determined TBI severity using criteria as suggested by Annegers et al.,[12] characterizing TBI as mild when the associated loss of consciousness or posttraumatic amnesia was less than 30 minutes in duration. Patients with longer duration of posttraumatic unconsciousness or amnesia, the presence of skull or radiographic evidence of TBI (based on conventional imaging modalities) were characterized as having moderate to severe TBI. These studies could be superficially interpreted as mild TBI (mTBI), being somehow more pathogenically associated with PNES. However, since PNES have been reported following TBIs of all severity levels (mild, moderate and severe),[10, 11] the observed distribution (87%) may simply mirror the overall incidence rate of mTBI, representing 80–90% of all head injury cases in the general population.[13] Within the past decade, significant advances in neuroimaging methods have uncovered macro- and submacroscopic abnormalities in patients with all severity levels of TBI (including mTBI) and/or PNES – findings which were previously not evident with conventional imaging modalities. Pertinent findings postulating the contribution of TBI to the neurobiological underpinnings of PNES will be further explored in this review.

Nascent literature pertaining to neuroimaging of PNES has shown divergent results, with different studies identifying varying potential regions of interest despite having study subjects from a similar population.[14] In view of these divergent results, this review will highlight notable regional substrates, as well as more widespread network abnormalities where key studies have converged to postulate the neurobiological overlap between TBI and PNES.

The uncinate fasciculus (UF) is a white matter association tract that connects anterior temporal structures (e.g., amygdala, hippocampus) to prefrontal cortices (e.g., orbitofrontal cortex), and it has been directly implicated in psychiatric disorders.[15] More specifically, the temporo-amygdala-orbitofrontal network has been hypothesized to be critically involved in integration of emotional states with cognition and behavior.[16] Notably, a diffusion tensor imaging (DTI) study showed that the UF is affected in 29% of 34 patients who sustained mTBI.[17] Applying DTI methods to patients with patients with PNES, one study observed abnormal DTI parameter (fractional anisotropy – FA) involving the left UF, superior temporal gyrus and subcortical structures when compared to healthy controls.[18] Another DTI study found similar FA values between patients with PNES versus controls, but highlighted that patients with PNES demonstrated a significant asymmetry in the number of reconstructed UF streamlines (right greater than left). This asymmetry in UF streamlines was not exhibited in controls.[19] De novo PNES has been reported in case series after general neurosurgery[20] and systematically investigated after epilepsy surgery, affecting 2.4–8.8% of patients who had neurosurgery.[21-23] Most of epilepsy surgery cases entailed complete or partial resections for temporal lobe, frequently interrupting the UF and its limbic connections.

Among the major functional limbic networks, the UF exhibits high heritability as measured by degree of genetic variances between monozygotic and dizygotic twins.[24] The UF has also been characterized as having a protracted maturation process, undergoing developmental evolution well into the third decade of life.[25] In the aforementioned DTI study, an inverse correlation was observed between the degree of UF asymmetry and age at PNES onset (i.e., higher asymmetry indices were associated with younger ages at PNES onset).[18] A corollary to these observations could be that TBI at an earlier age (combined with inherited UF disturbance, when present) may contribute in parts to microstructural damage to the UF that confer vulnerability to later development of PNES. As such, TBI and genetic constitution could be considered as predisposing factors in the biopsychosocial etiologic model for PNES.

The default mode network (DMN) represents a brain network composed of the following nodes: rostral anterior cingulate gyrus, superior temporal and supramarginal gyrus, posterior cingulate gyrus and ventromedial prefrontal cortex.[26] The DMN subserves self-reflective mental activity and is more active at rest than during tasks requiring attention. Disruption of functional interactions within DMN after TBI was associated with impairment of both self-awareness[27] and inhibitory cognitive control.[28] A study utilizing high-density electroencephalography (EEG) found that PNES frequency correlated with degree of hypo-synchronization within the prefrontal and parietal regions, both of which are integral components of the DMN.[29]

A novel Integrative Cognitive Model (ICM) aims to bring together existing theories of PNES phenomenology toward a singular explanatory framework.[30] The ICM postulates that dysfunction of inhibitory processing represents a key late factor among a series of steps that precipitate PNES. This impairment of inhibitory control may potentially arise from disturbance within the DMN.[31] As such, TBI insulting critical brain substrates (e.g., DMN) could contribute in part as Precipitating factors in the biopsychosocial etiologic framework for PNES.

Recent studies of patients with PNES have utilized robust data-driven, functional connectivity analyses which investigate whole brain networks rather the pre-defined regions of interest (e.g., independent component analysis, graph theory). These advanced methods have demonstrated that in addition to changes within the DMN, more widespread alterations in fronto-parietal (attentional), emotional processing, executive control and sensorimotor networks.[32] Rather than a focal neuroanatomical process, these and other functional connectivity studies[33] advocate conceptualizing PNES as having disrupted neural networks, with seizure manifestations developing from alterations within, as well as abnormal interaction across, the aforementioned networks (Figure 10.2). Distinct disruptions to various parts of these involved networks may also contribute to the observed variations in PNES phenomenology.[34] These neural networks are thought to

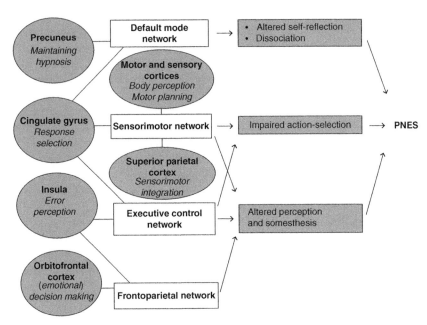

Figure 10.2 Conceptualization of psychogenic nonepileptic seizures as neural network disorder: Seizure manifestations develop from alterations within as well as abnormal interaction across key networks that contribute to altered self-reflection, dissociation, impaired action-selection and altered perception/somesthesis. From van der Kruijs et al.,[31] with permission.

represent recursive large-scale networks, typical of those involved with conscious awareness of sensory input and behavior (metacognitive processes).[31] Some have posited that metacognition is a unique process to humans, which may explain the lack of animal models of conversion disorder.[35] The long-range trajectory of the connectivity within such networks augments susceptibility to axonal shearing or straining forces from TBI, reflecting another plausible neuropathophysiological link between TBI and the development of dissociative symptoms accompanying PNES.[7]

Overall, the present literature in the neuroimaging of PNES is limited but growing, with early studies generally of small sample sizes that did not compare patients with PNES to controls matched for neuropsychiatric conditions. More studies comparing the overlap of network abnormalities evident in PNES with neuroanatomically based brain disorders (i.e., TBI) are needed. Further understanding of the neural basis behind the contribution of TBI to PNES does not negate or contradict the more commonly cited cognitive-behavioral mechanisms, but rather underscores the inextricable concurrence of multiple factors (structural, functional and psychological) as stipulated in the biopsychosocial framework for PNES. The psychological effects of TBI will be explored next.

Psychological Effects of TBI as Precipitating Factors

TBI, even at a mild degree, can induce significant level of stress and anxiety. About 14% of subjects who sustained mTBI from motor vehicle accident were diagnosed with acute stress disorder within 1 month of the injury.[36] Patients who sustained mTBI were likely to have ongoing symptoms at 12 months, compared to patients with orthopedic limb injuries.[37]

In predisposed individuals (including 80% of patients who experience acute stress disorder), stressors from the trauma can induce long-term changes in stress-responsivity and metacognitive function, ultimately fulfilling the diagnostic criteria for posttraumatic stress disorder (PTSD).[38] Moreover, several studies involving either civilians or veterans have highlighted the significant association of PTSD with the development of PNES.[2, 39, 40] Among US Veterans, PTSD was shown to significantly increase the likelihood of diagnosing PNES versus epileptic seizures when mTBI was the purported seizure etiology.[40] Based on these observations, investigators have inferred that PTSD may subserve a moderating role in the development of PNES, without which mTBI might be one-step away or entirely unrelated to PNES[7] (Figure 10.3). PTSD may also mediate the development of other somatic symptoms in Veterans who have sustained mTBI, including cognitive[41] and severity of postconcussive[42] symptoms.

Among patients who develop PTSD, some symptoms usually emerge within the first 3 months after the trauma. A subsequent delay of months or years (rarer, delayed expression PTSD) can transpire before DSM-5 criteria for the diagnosis are met.[1] Moreover, some investigators have conceptualized PNES as a manifestation of the dissociative subtype of

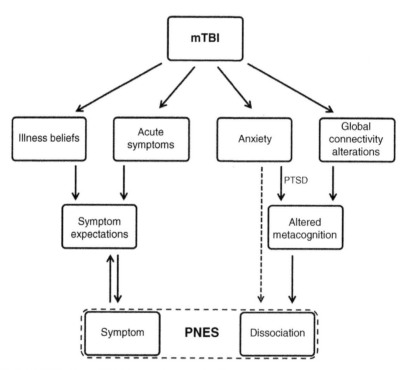

Figure 10.3 Mild TBI leading to PNES via several potential pathways. In predisposed individuals, trauma can induce long-term changes in stress responsivity and metacognition that define PTSD. In turn, PTSD could subserve a moderating role toward the development of PNES. Illness beliefs combined with anxious misattribution of acute symptoms (i.e., post-concussive symptoms) can foment maladaptive symptom modelling. Abbreviations: PNES, psychogenic nonepileptic seizures; TBI, traumatic brain injury; PTSD, postraumatic stress disorder. Modified from Popkirov et al.,[7] with permission.

PTSD.[43] Altogether, the expression of PTSD following TBI could be interpreted as a Precipitating factor in the biopsychosocial etiologic model for PNES.

Mild TBI frequently combines highly emotionally stressful situations (e.g., vehicular accidents and their aftermath, combat theater-related events) with acute neuropsychiatric dysfunction in motor/sensory faculties, memory and consciousness (e.g., post-concussive syndrome). Under such scenarios of heightened distress, illness beliefs regarding risk for posttraumatic epilepsy, combined with anxious misattribution of post-concussive symptoms can foment maladaptive symptom modelling – patient's own learnt mental representation of seizure symptoms and expectation of how seizures express[44] (Figure 10.3). When confronted with trauma reminders, unbearable stressors or unconscious emotional/somatic cues, PNES are triggered as part of a maladjusted emotional and physical stress response.[7, 45] Similar cognitive behavioral mechanisms have been proposed to instigate other non-PNES functional neurological disorders. In a systemic review of 869 patients with motor or sensory conversion symptoms, 37% had reported preceding physical injury.[46] Among 50 patients with psychogenic (functional) movement disorders (PMD), 22% experienced preceding physical injury typically involving the peripheral soft tissues.[47] In many of these reported cases, the demonstration of functional symptoms following brain-sparing traumatic injuries robustly support the cognitively and emotionally mediated effects of the physical traumas, independent of any neuronal disturbances within the brain.

An aforementioned study reported that 80% of patients reported the physical event within 3 months prior to onset of the PMD.[48] In addition, since maladaptive symptom modelling following TBI may subserve a role in the expression and triggering of PNES, it could be considered as a Precipitating factor in the biopsychosocial etiologic model for PNES.

TBI as a Perpetuating Factor

Compared to pre-injury, patients with mTBI have shown higher prevalence of comorbid psychiatric disorder post-injury, particularly with regards to novel onset of depression and personality disorders.[49, 50] By contributing to novel onset of psychiatric disorders post-injury, it is conceivable that mTBI could adversely impact PNES outcome by subserving a perpetuating role.

The literature that examines the impact of TBI upon the clinical outcomes of patients with PNES is sparse. One cross-sectional study compared the psychiatric and functioning outcome measures of 41 patients with history of PNES and TBI (P + T) versus 51 patients with PNES but no TBI (P − T). When compared to those with P − T, patients with P + T showed significantly increased odds of having major depression, impulsivity (a cluster B personality trait), PTSD and a trauma/abuse history.[51] Patients with P + T also had significantly lower mean Global Assessment of Functioning (GAF) scores and showed disability rates about twice of those with P − T.[51] The retrospective nature of this study limits inference regarding causation (i.e., TBI directly causing heightened comorbidities in patients with PNES). Thirteen of the 41 patients with P + T had the TBI after the onset of PNES. An alternative consideration may be that for some patients with PNES, the observed heightened comorbidities existed beforehand and contributed to TBI-prone behaviors that resulted in the subsequent TBI. Furthermore, the observed result may also potentially arise from a combined/synergistic effect of TBI and PNES.[51] Nevertheless, while limited, there is evidence that TBI can contribute to psychiatric comorbidities/outcomes in patients with PNES and in turn represents a Perpetuating factor in the biopsychosocial etiologic framework for PNES.

Conclusion

By illustrating how TBI may subserve Predisposing, Precipitating and Perpetuating roles in the development of PNES, this review underscores the concurrence of multiple factors (structural, functional and psychological) as stipulated in the biopsychosocial etiologic framework for PNES. At the same time, limitations of the current literature, particularly as pertaining to studies that compare the overlap of network abnormalities observed in PNES with neuroanatomically based brain disorders, and studies evaluating the impact of TBI upon the clinical outcomes of patients with PNES have been highlighted. Further investigations in these areas may promote a more comprehensive understanding of PNES development/perpetuation and in turn may help devise treatment strategies.

References

1. American Psychiatric Association. *Diagnostic and Statistical Manual of Mental Disorders*, fifth edition (DSM-5). Washington, DC : American Psychiatric Association, 2013.

2. Bowman ES, Markand ON. Psychodynamics and psychiatric diagnoses of pseudoseizure subjects. *Am J Psychiatry* 1996;153:57–63.

3. LaFrance Jr WC, Bjønaes H. Chapter 28. Designing Treatment Plans Based on Etiology of Psychogenic Noenpileptic Seizures. In: LaFrance Jr WC, Schachter SC, editors. *Gates and Rowan's Nonepileptic Seizures*. 4th ed. New York: Cambridge University Press; 2018. p. 283–99.

4. LaFrance WC, Jr. , Devinsky O. Treatment of nonepileptic seizures. *Epilepsy Behav* 2002;3(5 Supplement 1): S19–23.

5. LaFrance WC, Jr, Barry JJ. Update on treatments of psychological nonepileptic seizures. *Epilepsy Behav* 2005;7:364–74.

6. Reuber M. The etiology of psychogenic non-epileptic seizures: toward a biopsychosocial model. *Neurol Clin* 2009;27:909–24.

7. Popkirov S, Carson AJ, Stone J. Scared or scarred: Could 'dissociogenic' lesions predispose to nonepileptic seizures after head trauma? *Seizure* 2018;8:127–32.

8. Benbadis SR, Allen Hauser W. An estimate of the prevalence of psychogenic non-epileptic seizures. *Seizure* 2000;9:280–1.

9. Frost RB, Farrer TJ, Primosch M, Hedges DW. Prevalence of traumatic brain injury in the general adult population: a meta-analysis. *Neuroepidemiology* 2013;40:154–9.

10. Salinsky M, Storzbach D, Goy E, Evrard C. Traumatic brain injury and psychogenic seizures in veterans. *J Head Trauma Rehabil* 2015;30:E65–70.

11. Hudak AM, Trivedi K, Harper CR, *et al.* Evaluation of seizure-like episodes in survivors of moderate and severe traumatic brain injury. *J Head Trauma Rehabil* 2004;19:290–5.

12. Annegers JF, Hauser WA, Coan SP, Rocca WA. A population-based study of seizures after traumatic brain injuries. *N Engl J Med* 1998;338:20–4.

13. Blennow K, Brody DL, Kochanek PM, *et al.* Traumatic brain injuries. *Nat Rev Dis Primers* 2016;17;2:16084.

14. Szaflarski JP, LaFrance WC Jr. Psychogenic nonepileptic seizures (PNES) as a network disorder – evidence from neuroimaging of functional (psychogenic) neurological disorders. *Epilepsy Curr* 2018;18:211–16.

15. Alnæs D, Kaufmann T, Doan NT, *et al.* Association of heritable cognitive ability and psychopathology with white matter

properties in children and adolescents. *JAMA Psychiatry* 2018;75:287–95.

16. Von Der Heide RJ, Skipper LM, Klobusicky E, Olson IR. Dissecting the uncinate fasciculus: disorders, controversies and a hypothesis. *Brain* 2013;136: 1692–707.

17. Niogi SN, Mukherjee P, Ghajar J, et al. Extent of microstructural white matter injury in postconcussive syndrome correlates with impaired cognitive reaction time: a 3 T diffusion tensor imaging study of mild traumatic brain injury. *Am J Neuroradiol.* 2008;29:967–73.

18. Lee S, Allendorfer JB, Gaston TE, et al. White matter diffusion abnormalities in patients with psychogenic non-epileptic seizures. *Brain Res* 2015;1620:169–76.

19. Hernando KA, Szaflarski JP, Ver Hoef LW, Lee S, Allendorfer JB. Uncinate fasciculus connectivity in patients with psychogenic nonepileptic seizures: A preliminary diffusion tensor tractography study. *Epilepsy Behav* 2015, 5:68–73.

20. Reuber M, Kral T, Kurthen M, Elger CE. New-onset psychogenic seizures after intracranial neurosurgery. *Acta Neurochir (Wien)* 2002;44:901–7.

21. Asadi-Pooya AA, Asadollahi M, Tinker J, Nei M, Sperling MR. Post-epilepsy surgery psychogenic nonepileptic seizures. *Epilepsia* 2016;57:1691–6.

22. Ney GC, Barr WB, Napolitano C, Decker R, Schaul N. New-onset psychogenic seizures after surgery for epilepsy. *Arch Neurol* 1998;5:726–30.

23. Glosser G, Roberts D, Glosser DS. Nonepileptic seizures after resective epilepsy surgery. *Epilepsia* 1999;40:1750–4.

24. Budisavljevic S, Kawadler JM, Dell'Acqua F, et al. Heritability of the limbic networks. *Soc Cogn Affect Neurosci* 2016;11:746–57.

25. Lebel C, Gee M, Camicioli R, Wieler M, Martin W, Beaulieu C. Diffusion tensor imaging of white matter tract evolution over the lifespan. *Neuroimage* 2012;60:340–52.

26. Greicius MD, Krasnow B, Reiss AL, Menon V. Functional connectivity in the resting brain: a network analysis of the default mode hypothesis. *Proc Natl Acad Sci U S A* 2003;100:253–8.

27. Ham TE, Bonnelle V, Hellyer P, et al. The neural basis of impaired self-awareness after traumatic brain injury. *Brain* 2014;137:586–97.

28. Bonnelle V, Ham TE, Leech R, et al. Salience network integrity predicts default mode network function after traumatic brain injury. *Proc Natl Acad Sci U S A* 2012;109:4690–5.

29. Knyazeva MG, Jalili M, Frackowiak RS, Rossetti AO. Psychogenic seizures and frontal disconnection: EEG synchronisation study. *J Neurol Neurosurg Psychiatry* 2011;82:505–11.

30. Reuber M, Brown RJ. Understanding psychogenic nonepileptic seizures-Phenomenology, semiology and the Integrative Cognitive Model. *Seizure* 2017;4:199–205.

31. van der Kruijs SJ, Jagannathan SR, Bodde NM, et al. Resting-state networks and dissociation in psychogenic non-epileptic seizures. *J Psychiatr Res* 2014;54:126–33.

32. Ding J, An D, Liao W, Wu G, Xu Q, Zhou D, Chen H. Abnormal functional connectivity density in psychogenic non-epileptic seizures. *Epilepsy Res* 2014;108:1184–94.

33. Ding JR, An D, Liao W, et al. Altered functional and structural connectivity networks in psychogenic non-epileptic seizures. *PLoS One* 2013;8:e63850.

34. Li R, Li Y, An D, Gong Q, Zhou D, Chen H. Altered regional activity and inter-regional functional connectivity in psychogenic non-epileptic seizures. *Sci Rep* 2015;5:11635.

35. Cretton A, Brown RJ, LaFrance WC, Jr., Aybek S. What does neuroscience tell us about the conversion model of functional neurological disorders? *J Neuropsychiatry Clin Neurosci.* 2019:32:24–32.

36. Li R, Liu K, Ma X, *et al.* Altered functional connectivity patterns of the insular subregions in psychogenic nonepileptic seizures. *Brain Topogr* 2015;28:636–45.

37. Nelson LD, Temkin NR, Dikmen S, et al. Recovery after mild traumatic brain injury in patients presenting to US Level I Trauma Centers: A Transforming Research and Clinical Knowledge in Traumatic Brain Injury (TRACK-TBI) study. *JAMA Neurology* 2019:76:1049–59.

38. Voon V, Cavanna AE, Coburn K, Sampson S, Reeve A, LaFrance WC Jr. Functional neuroanatomy and neurophysiology of functional neurological disorders (conversion disorder). *J Neuropsychiatry Clin Neurosci* 2016;28:168–9.

39. Sergent C, Dehaene S. Neural processes underlying conscious perception: experimental findings and a global neuronal workspace framework. *J Physiol Paris* 2004;98:374–84.

40. Harvey AG, Bryant RA. Acute stress disorder after mild traumatic brain injury. *J Nerv Ment Dis* 1998;186:333–7.

41. Harvey AG, Bryant RA. Two-year prospective evaluation of the relationship between acute stress disorder and posttraumatic stress disorder following mild traumatic brain injury. *Am J Psychiatry* 2000;157:626–8.

42. Salinsky M, Evrard C, Storzbach D, Pugh MJ. Psychiatric comorbidity in veterans with psychogenic seizures. *Epilepsy Behav* 2012;25:345–9.

43. Rosenberg HJ, Rosenberg SD, Williamson PD, Wolford GL 2nd. A comparative study of trauma and posttraumatic stress disorder prevalence in epilepsy patients and psychogenic nonepileptic seizure patients. *Epilepsia* 2000;41:447–52.

44. Spencer RJ, Drag LL, Walker SJ, Bieliauskas LA. Self-reported cognitive symptoms following mild traumatic brain injury are poorly associated with neuropsychological performance in OIF/OEF veterans. *J Rehabil Res Dev* 2010;47:521–30.

45. Lippa SM, Pastorek NJ, Benge JF, Thornton GM. Postconcussive symptoms after blast and nonblast-related mild traumatic brain injuries in Afghanistan and Iraq war veterans. *J Int Neuropsychol Soc* 2010;16:856–66.

46. Fiszman A, Alves-Leon SV, Nunes RG, D'Andrea I, Figueira I. Traumatic events and posttraumatic stress disorder in patients with psychogenic nonepileptic seizures: a critical review. *Epilepsy Behav* 2004;5:818–25.

47. Stone J, Carson A, Aditya H, *et al.* The role of physical injury in motor and sensory conversion symptoms: a systematic and narrative review. *J Psychosom Res* 2009;66:383–90.

48. Pareés I, Kojovic M, Pires C, *et al.* Physical precipitating factors in functional movement disorders. *J Neurol Sci* 2014;338 (1–2):174–7.

49. Whelan-Goodinson R, Ponsford J, Johnston L, Grant F. Psychiatric disorders following traumatic brain injury: their nature and frequency. *J Head Trauma Rehabil* 2009;24:324–32.

50. Hibbard MR, Bogdany J, Uysal S, *et al.* Axis II psychopathology in individuals with traumatic brain injury. *Brain Inj* 2000;14:45–61.

51. LaFrance WC Jr, Deluca M, Machan JT, Fava JL. Traumatic brain injury and psychogenic nonepileptic seizures yield worse outcomes. *Epilepsia* 2013;54:718–25.

Post-traumatic Epilepsy and Post-traumatic Stress Disorder

Marco Mula

Introduction

The intersection between post-traumatic stress disorder (PTSD) and traumatic brain injury (TBI) has become increasingly important during the last few years, especially in the context of military medicine.[1, 2]

In 2013, the American Psychiatric Association revised the diagnostic criteria for PTSD in the fifth edition of its *Diagnostic and Statistical Manual of Mental Disorders* (DSM-5).[3] In DSM-5, PTSD is not classified among anxiety disorders anymore because it is now included in a new category named 'Trauma- and Stressor-Related Disorders'. One of the novel aspects of the new classification is that all conditions included in this group require exposure to a traumatic or stressful event as a diagnostic criterion.

Traumatic and stressful events are not infrequent but epidemiological studies show that only a minority of people exposed to a traumatic stressor develop PTSD. Data from the National Comorbidity Survey have shown that around 1 in 8 woman and fewer than 1 in 10 men develop PTSD after a trauma.[4, 5] It seems established that the severity of the trauma, in physical and psychological terms, is one of the main determinants for the development of PTSD. For example, 55% of rape victims develop PTSD against only 7.5% of accident victims.[6] In this context, the relationship between PTSD and TBI is particularly fascinating. In the past, PTSD was considered rare in TBI because the loss of consciousness at the time of the trauma was thought to prevent the encoding of potentially traumatic memories which are necessary for the development of PTSD.[7] On the contrary, cumulating evidence has subsequently challenged this concept showing that PTSD can follow any TBI from mild to severe[8] and patients can suffer episodes of more or less prolonged retrograde and anterograde amnesia, sometimes with no recollection of the traumatic experience itself.[6] But what is the relationship between PTSD, TBI and post-traumatic epilepsy (PTE)? The aim of this chapter is to discuss the relationships between PTSD and epilepsy in terms of epidemiology, neurobiological mechanisms and phenomenology. A pragmatic approach to the treatment of PTSD in epilepsy is also presented.

Neurobiology

The neurobiology of PTSD is complex and only partially overlaps with that of anxiety disorder. In fact, as compared to anxiety disorders, PTSD is characterized by a number of immune, endocrine, inflammatory and epigenetic changes which seem to be related to the exposure to a stressor[9] and some of them can be potentially relevant in the comorbidity between PTSD and epilepsy.

Table 11.1 Neurobiological mechanisms implicated in PTSD that may be of relevance in epilepsy

A: Neurochemical level
Increased CRH levels
Decreased serotonin levels
Decreased GABA activity
Increased NMDA activity

B: Neuroanatomical level
Reduced hippocampal volumes
Increased amygdala firing
Reduced prefrontal cortex volumes
Reduced anterior cingulate volumes

A core feature of PTSD is the dysfunction of the hypothalamic–pituitary–adrenal axis driven by sustained high levels of corticotropin-releasing hormone (CRH).[10] High CRH levels are responsible for adrenocorticotrophin desensitization to CRH stimulation that ultimately leads to abnormal cortisol responses to stress and chronic hypocortisolism.[10] Although the chronic hypocortisolism may sound like a paradox, it is, on the contrary, a basic principle of PTSD as these patients present with abnormal stress reactivity due to a decreased availability of stress hormones.

High CRH levels are a potential key factor explaining the link between PTSD and epilepsy (Table 11.1). In fact, high CRH levels are associated with progressive neuronal and volume loss in the hippocampi[11] as well as hippocampal downregulation of GABA-A receptors[12] and upregulation of NMDA receptors in the prefrontal cortex.[10]. All these changes are widely described in people with temporal lobe epilepsy and may contribute to the bidirectional relationship suggested by epidemiological studies in the subsequent section.

Another core feature of PTSD is the abnormal regulation of a number of neurotransmitters especially catecholamines and serotonin.[10] The chronically high dopamine and noradrenalin levels are responsible for hyperarousal symptoms, increased blood pressure and heart rates but also increased encoding of fear memories.[13] This seems also to be associated with a progressive downregulation of 5HT1A receptors and a progressive reduction of serotonin levels.[14] The low serotonin levels would ultimately be responsible for the intrusive memories, the impulsivity and the hypervigilance described in patients with PTSD. However, low serotonin levels have been also described in animal models of epilepsy such as genetically epilepsy-prone rats, the pilocarpine status epilepticus model in Wistar rats and rhesus monkeys,[15] further supporting the link between PTSD and epilepsy.

Epidemiology

Data from the World Mental Health survey showed lifetime prevalence rates for PTSD in Europe ranging from 2% of Italy and Spain to 8.8% of Northern Ireland while data from the US Department of Veterans Affairs, National Centre for PTSD, reported lifetime prevalence rates among adult Americans of about 6.8%.[16]

Data about the prevalence of PTSD in epilepsy are limited. A US study in 174 patients using the Mini-International Neuropsychiatric Interview (MINI) reported a diagnosis of current (active) PTSD in 5.7% of patients[17] but a meta-analysis of 27 studies of anxiety disorders involving more than 3,000 people with epilepsy showed a pooled prevalence of 0.09% (95%CI 0.05–1.8).[18] The conflicting results probably reflect variations in individual subpopulations of patients with epilepsy. For example, data from a multicentre study of US Veterans showed prevalence rates for PTSD in PTE in the region of 13%.[19] It is, therefore, evident that the prevalence of PTSD is also influenced by the specific aetiology of the epilepsy, being higher in people with PTE as compared to other aetiologies (e.g. vascular, cortical dysplasia or hippocampal sclerosis) or other epilepsy syndromes (e.g. focal vs. generalized). However, data on the prevalence of PTSD in relationship to the specific epilepsy syndrome are still lacking.

A number of studies have shown a bidirectional relationship between epilepsy and depression, meaning that not only epilepsy is burdened by an increased prevalence of depression but also depression is associated with an increased risk of developing epilepsy.[20] The same relationship has been established also for a number of other psychiatric disorders, from autism and attention deficit hyperactivity disorder to schizophrenia and other thought disorders. Data on the relationship between PTSD and epilepsy are almost non-existent with a single study available. A US study in veterans older than 65 shows that a previous history of anxiety disorders (at the time of this study PTSD was listed among anxiety disorders) is significantly more common in those who developed epilepsy as compared to controls.[21] A cohort Danish study involving more than 200,000 subjects showed that people on selective serotonin reuptake inhibitors (SSRIs) at the time of the TBI are 5.6 times more likely to develop epilepsy than those who were not on SSRIs.[22] Given that previous studies have shown that SSRIs per se are not associated with an increased risk of seizures,[23] it is possible to speculate that to be on SSRI is likely to represent an indicator of a mood or anxiety disorder severe enough to require pharmacological treatment. A large cross-sectional study from Taiwan, using data from the Health Insurance Database and including more than 6,000 individuals, showed that people with PTSD have a 3–6 times increased risk of developing epilepsy after adjusting for demographic, medical and psychiatric comorbidities.[24] All these data taken together seem to suggest that the relationship between PTSD and epilepsy is possibly similar to that shown for other psychiatric conditions.

Clinical Implications

In people with epilepsy, psychiatric comorbidities have been historically associated with poor quality of life, but there are now data suggesting their role as a prognostic factor. In fact, psychiatric comorbidities are associated with a high risk of side effects from antiepileptic drugs, especially cognitive complaints and psychiatric side effects.[25] Psychiatric disorders are also associated with a 4-time increased risk of drug resistance in focal[26] and generalized epilepsies.[27] Psychiatric comorbidities are also associated with premature mortality,[28] and this may be due to a variety of reasons, including increased risk of substance or alcohol abuse, increased risk of injuries and increased suicide rates.

Data from a population-based study of over 57,000 people in Sweden showed that females with epilepsy and psychiatric disorders have a 5-fold increased risk of sudden unexpected death in epilepsy (SUDEP) compared to those without such comorbidities.[29]

Data on the specific role of PTSD in epilepsy are not available and further studies are needed in order to clarify whether PTSD is associated with a poor prognosis in people with PTE.

As already discussed in Chapter 10, PTSD and TBI are also strictly interlinked with psychogenic non-epileptic seizures (PNES). A retrospective study from the Veterans Affairs Medical Centre reported a 57% prevalence of PNES after TBI against a 35% of PTE.[30] Patients with PNES after TBI showed a strong correlation with a diagnosis of PTSD.[19] However, there are no specific data about the co-occurrence of PTE and PNES. A recent meta-analysis on the prevalence of PNES in people with epilepsy showed a pooled prevalence of 12%, while the prevalence of epilepsy in people with PNES was reported as high as 22%.[31] Given the strong association between TBI and PNES it is possible to speculate that the comorbidity between PTE and PNES could be substantial. However, it is important to point out that PNES seem to be more common in mild TBI while PTE is probably more common in moderate to severe TBI. Therefore, it may not be necessarily true that patients with PTE present higher PNES comorbidity rates than other epilepsy syndromes. The presence of PTSD may represent a valuable clinical indicator to investigate further the relationship among these clinical entities.

Management of PTSD in Epilepsy

There are no data on the treatment of PTSD in the context of epilepsy and this reflects the paucity of data about the management of anxiety disorders in epilepsy.[32] In such a case, it seems reasonable to adapt current guidelines of treatment used outside epilepsy to the specific needs of people with epilepsy including interactions and seizure risk.

Psychological Interventions

It is now established that trauma-focused cognitive behavioural therapy (CBT) and eye movement desensitization and reprocessing (EMDR) are both effective in PTSD and superior to stress management.[33]

Studies comparing psychological and pharmacological interventions are limited. However, a number of small studies have shown the advantages of a combined treatment.[34]

Pharmacological Treatments

Regarding the acute treatment, data from randomized placebo-controlled trials (RCTs) suggest that most antidepressants, including SSRIs, are effective in PTSD.[35] However, a meta-analysis of 37 RCTs using structured scales showed evidence only for paroxetine, sertraline and venlafaxine.[36] Apart from antidepressants, there seems to be some evidence for the antipsychotics risperidone and olanzapine and the anticonvulsant topiramate.[35] Medications which failed RCTs include citalopram, alprazolam, tiagabine and valproate.[35]

Prospective studies investigating the long-term treatment of PTSD are limited and most of the longitudinal data come from retrospective studies. Available data suggest that around 50% of patients with PTSD experiences a chronic course of the disease but the proportion of patients responding to treatment also increases over time.[36, 37] The number of studies focusing on relapse prevention is scant with only a few RCTs available supporting evidence for fluoxetine[38] and sertraline.[39]

Drug Interactions and Seizure Risk

When treating PTSD in people with epilepsy, clinicians need to pay attention to interactions with antiepileptic drugs and the potential effect of psychotropic medications on the seizure threshold (Table 11.2).

Table 11.2 Pharmacological management of PTSD in epilepsy

First line	First choice: Sertraline
	Second: Venlafaxine or paroxetine
Augmentation strategies	First choice: Topiramate
	Second: Risperidone
	Third: Olanzapine

Regarding antidepressants, data from unselected samples of patients with epilepsy suggest that sertraline is not associated with significant drug–drug interactions and there is no evidence of seizure worsening.

It is established that first generation of antiepileptic drugs like carbamazepine (CBZ), phenytoin (PHT) and barbiturates are powerful inducers of drug-metabolizing enzymes including the cytochrome P450 (CYP) and the glucuronosyltransferase (UGT) systems while valproate (VPA) is a broad spectrum enzyme inhibitor.[40, 41] The CYP and UGT systems contribute to the metabolism of all antidepressants and, for this reason all first generation antiepileptic drugs may have interactions with antidepressants. CBZ, PHT and barbiturates seem to reduce the plasma levels of SSRIs and serotonin–norepinephrine reuptake inhibitors (SNRIs) by at least 25% but whether this is clinically relevant depends on the individual patient.[40, 41] Studies on VPA are limited but it seems that there are no clinically relevant pharmacokinetic interactions with SSRIs or SNRIs.[40, 41] As far as other antidepressants, tricyclic antidepressants have a complex metabolism mediated by the CYP and the UGT systems and they represent complex drugs to be used in polytherapy especially with first generation antiepileptic drugs. For this reason, clinical monitoring and dose adjustment according to clinical response are always recommended.

Compared to first generation compounds, second and third generation antiepileptic drugs have a better pharmacokinetic profile with a low risk for interactions. Oxcarbazepine and topiramate are the only ones which may have weak inducing properties at high doses but systematic studies on the clinical relevance of such an effect are lacking.

Clinicians are often concerned by the potential risk of seizures with antidepressants. However, this was based on an *a priori* assumption rather than on clinical evidence.[40] The issue of drug-related seizures is quite complex and it does not involve only psychotropic medications as it has been described with a number of other drugs.[42] In general terms, multiple factors have to be taken into account and studies in animal models suggest that serotonin potentiation may even be anticonvulsant.[43] Among all antidepressants, a clear association with seizures has been established only for maprotiline, high doses of clomipramine and amitriptyline (>200 mg), high doses of bupropion in the immediate release formulation (>450 mg).[40] For all other antidepressants, there is no clear evidence of an increased risk of seizures. A systematic review of data from placebo-controlled trials with psychotropic drugs, submitted to the United States Federal Drug Administration (FDA), shows that that the frequency of seizures with SSRIs is even lower than placebo.[23] In addition, if we take into account that patients with depression or anxiety disorders have an increased risk of seizures, the reported prevalence of seizures during treatment with SSRIs is even lower than expected, suggesting SSRIs reduce the risk of seizures.[40] It is anyway important to bear in mind that current knowledge on seizure prevalence during antidepressant drug treatment is based on psychiatric populations, and it is still unknown whether these data can be transferred to patients with epilepsy and whether some epileptic syndromes are more at risk than others.

Regarding antipsychotic drugs, available data suggest that risperidone is safest option in terms of interaction and seizure risk.[44] Clozapine has the highest risk of seizures when compared to placebo with a standardized incident ratio of 9.5.[23] Olanzapine and quetiapine carry also some risk but to a lesser extent, while all other antipsychotics are no different from placebo.[23] A large community-based Taiwanese study involving 288,397 people showed that second generation antipsychotics like risperidone and aripiprazole have an even lower risk of seizures than first generation drugs like chlorprothixene, thioridazine and haloperidol.[45]

References

1. Jindal RM. Refugees, asylum seekers, and immigrants in clinical trials. *Lancet* 2020;395:30–1.

2. Charlson F, van Ommeren M, Flaxman A, Cornett J, Whiteford H, Saxena S. New WHO prevalence estimates of mental disorders in conflict settings: a systematic review and meta-analysis. *Lancet* 2019;394:240–8.

3. Association AP. *Diagnostic and Statistical Manual of Mental Disorders*, Fifth Edition. 5th edition. Washington, DC: American Psychiatric Publishing; 2013.

4. Breslau N, Davis GC, Andreski P, Peterson E. Traumatic events and posttraumatic stress disorder in an urban population of young adults. *Arch Gen Psychiatry* 1991;48:216–22.

5. Kessler RC, Sonnega A, Bromet E, Hughes M, Nelson CB. Posttraumatic stress disorder in the National Comorbidity Survey. *Arch Gen Psychiatry* 1995;52:1048–60.

6. Bryant R. Post-traumatic stress disorder vs traumatic brain injury. *Dialogues Clin Neurosci* 2011;13:251–62.

7. Price KP. Posttraumatic stress disorder and concussion: Are they incompatible? *Defense Law Journal* 1994;43: 113–20.

8. Bryant RA, Harvey AG. Relationship between acute stress disorder and posttraumatic stress disorder following mild traumatic brain injury. *Am J Psychiatry* 1998;155:625–9.

9. Shalev A, Liberzon I, Marmar C. Post-traumatic stress disorder. *N Engl J Med* 2017;376:2459–69.

10. Sherin JE, Nemeroff CB. Post-traumatic stress disorder: the neurobiological impact of psychological trauma. *Dialogues Clin Neurosci* 2011;13:263–78.

11. Bremner JD, Elzinga B, Schmahl C, Vermetten E. Structural and functional plasticity of the human brain in posttraumatic stress disorder. *Prog Brain Res* 2008;167:171–86.

12. Geuze E, van Berckel BNM, Lammertsma AA, et al. Reduced GABAA benzodiazepine receptor binding in veterans with post-traumatic stress disorder. *Mol Psychiatry* 2008;13:74–83, 3.

13. Strawn JR, Geracioti TD. Noradrenergic dysfunction and the psychopharmacology of posttraumatic stress disorder. *Depress Anxiety* 2008;25:260–71.

14. Vermetten E, Bremner JD. Circuits and systems in stress. II. Applications to neurobiology and treatment in posttraumatic stress disorder. *Depress Anxiety* 2002;16:14–38.

15. Kanner AM. Can neurobiological pathogenic mechanisms of depression facilitate the development of seizure disorders? *Lancet Neurol* 2012 ;11:1093–102.

16. Atwoli L, Stein DJ, Koenen KC, McLaughlin KA. Epidemiology of posttraumatic stress disorder: prevalence, correlates and consequences. *Curr Opin Psychiatry* 2015;28:307–11.

17. Jones JE, Hermann BP, Barry JJ, Gilliam F, Kanner AM, Meador KJ. Clinical assessment of Axis I psychiatric morbidity in chronic epilepsy: a multicenter investigation. *J Neuropsychiatry Clin Neurosci* 2005;17:172–9.

18. Scott AJ, Sharpe L, Hunt C, Gandy M. Anxiety and depressive disorders in people with epilepsy: A meta-analysis. *Epilepsia* 2017;58:973–82.

19. Salinsky M, Rutecki P, Parko K, et al. Psychiatric comorbidity and traumatic brain injury attribution in patients with psychogenic nonepileptic or epileptic seizures: A multicenter study of US veterans. *Epilepsia* 2018;59:1945–53.

20. Mula M. Depression in epilepsy. *Curr Opin Neurol* 2017;30:180–6.

21. Ettinger AB, Copeland LA, Zeber JE, Van Cott AC, Pugh MJV. Are psychiatric disorders independent risk factors for new-onset epilepsy in older individuals? *Epilepsy Behav* 2010;17:70–4.

22. Christensen J, Pedersen HS, Fenger-Grøn M, Fann JR, Jones NC, Vestergaard M. Selective serotonin reuptake inhibitors and risk of epilepsy after traumatic brain injury – A population based cohort study. *PLoS ONE* 2019;14:e0219137.

23. Alper K, Schwartz KA, Kolts RL, Khan A. Seizure incidence in psychopharmacological clinical trials: an analysis of Food and Drug Administration (FDA) summary basis of approval reports. *Biol Psychiatry* 2007;62:345–54.

24. Chen Y-H, Wei H-T, Bai Y-M, et al. Risk of epilepsy in individuals with posttraumatic stress disorder: A nationwide longitudinal study. *Psychosom Med* 2017;79:664–9.

25. Stephen LJ, Wishart A, Brodie MJ. Psychiatric side effects and antiepileptic drugs: Observations from prospective audits. *Epilepsy Behav* 2017;71(Pt A):73–8.

26. Nogueira MH, Yasuda CL, Coan AC, Kanner AM, Cendes F. Concurrent mood and anxiety disorders are associated with pharmacoresistant seizures in patients with MTLE. *Epilepsia.* 2017;58:1268–76.

27. Stevelink R, Koeleman BPC, Sander JW, sen FE, Braun KPJ. Refractory juvenile myoclonic epilepsy: a meta-analysis of prevalence and risk factors. *Eur J Neurol* 2018;26:856–64.

28. Fazel S, Wolf A, Långström N, Newton CR, Lichtenstein P. Premature mortality in epilepsy and the role of psychiatric comorbidity: a total population study. *Lancet.* 2013;382:1646–54.

29. Sveinsson O, Andersson T, Carlsson S, Tomson T. The incidence of SUDEP: A nationwide population-based cohort study. *Neurology.* 2017 11;89:170–7.

30. Salinsky M, Storzbach D, Goy E, Evrard C. Traumatic brain injury and psychogenic seizures in veterans. *J Head Trauma Rehabil.* 2015;30:E65–70.

31. Kutlubaev MA, Xu Y, Hackett ML, Stone J. Dual diagnosis of epilepsy and psychogenic nonepileptic seizures: Systematic review and meta-analysis of frequency, correlates, and outcomes. *Epilepsy Behav.* 2018;89:70–8.

32. Mula M. Pharmacological treatment of anxiety disorders in adults with epilepsy. *Expert Opin Pharmacother.* 2018;19 (17):1867–74.

33. Bisson J, Andrew M. Psychological treatment of post-traumatic stress disorder (PTSD). *Cochrane Database Syst Rev* 2007 18;:CD003388.

34. Hetrick SE, McKenzie JE, Cox GR, Simmons MB, Merry SN. Newer generation antidepressants for depressive disorders in children and adolescents. *Cochrane Database Syst Rev* 2012 14;11: CD004851.

35. Baldwin DS, Anderson IM, Nutt DJ, et al. Evidence-based pharmacological treatment of anxiety disorders, post-traumatic stress disorder and obsessive-compulsive disorder: a revision of the 2005 guidelines from the British Association for Psychopharmacology. *J Psychopharmacol (Oxford).* 2014;28:403–39.

36. Ipser JC, Stein DJ. Evidence-based pharmacotherapy of post-traumatic stress disorder (PTSD).

Int J Neuropsychopharmacol 2012;15:825–40.

37. Davidson JRT. Pharmacologic treatment of acute and chronic stress following trauma: 2006. *J Clin Psychiatry* 2006;67 Suppl 2:34–9.

38. Martenyi F, Brown EB, Zhang H, Prakash A, Koke SC. Fluoxetine versus placebo in posttraumatic stress disorder. *J Clin Psychiatry* 2002;63:199–206.

39. Davidson JR, Payne VM, Connor KM, et al. Trauma, resilience and saliostasis: effects of treatment in post-traumatic stress disorder. *Int Clin Psychopharmacol* 2005;20:43–8.

40. Mula M. The pharmacological management of psychiatric comorbidities in patients with epilepsy. *Pharmacol Res* 2016;107:147–53.

41. Spina E, Pisani F, de Leon J. Clinically significant pharmacokinetic drug interactions of antiepileptic drugs with new antidepressants and new antipsychotics. *Pharmacol Res* 2016;106:72–86.

42. Ruffmann C, Bogliun G, Beghi E. Epileptogenic drugs: a systematic review. *Expert Rev Neurother* 2006;6:575–89.

43. Hamid H, Kanner AM. Should antidepressant drugs of the selective serotonin reuptake inhibitor family be tested as antiepileptic drugs? *Epilepsy Behav.* 2013;26:261–5.

44. Agrawal N, Mula M. Treatment of psychoses in patients with epilepsy: an update. *Ther Adv Psychopharmacol* 2019;9:2045125319862968.

45. Wu C-S, Wang S-C, Yeh I-J, Liu S-K. Comparative risk of seizure with use of first- and second-generation antipsychotics in patients with schizophrenia and mood disorders. *J Clin Psychiatry* 2016;77: e573–79.

Antiepileptogenic Therapies for Post-traumatic Epilepsy: Is There Any Evidence?

Francesco Brigo and Simona Lattanzi

Introduction

Traumatic brain injury (TBI) is a clinically heterogeneous condition, ranging from mild to severe forms, and represents one of the most common causes of acquired epilepsy, particularly among adults and elderly patients. The overall incidence of post-traumatic seizures in developed countries ranges from 4 to 53%[1]; this rather imprecise estimate is due to the high heterogeneity of studies, which differ for a variety of variables, including age of patients, severity of trauma, length of follow-up and often do not differentiate between early and late post-traumatic seizures.

Post-traumatic epilepsy accounts for approximately 20% of symptomatic epilepsy in the general population[2] and should be classified as a structural epilepsy.[3] Epileptic seizures may develop even several years after the head injury, and their occurrence depends mainly on the severity of the trauma. An epidemiological study has shown that the cumulative risk of developing post-traumatic seizures within 5 years from the event is 0.5% among patients with mild, 1.2% in those with moderate and 10% in those with severe TBI.[4]

After briefly discussing the differences between early (acute symptomatic) and late (unprovoked) post-traumatic seizures, with a focus on the underlying pathophysiology and long-term risk of seizure recurrence, this chapter will discuss the methodological issues and challenges of antiepileptogenesis trials and the role of antiepileptic drugs (AEDs) and neuroprotective agents in preventing post-traumatic seizures. Although animal studies have reported successful attempts to halt the process of epileptogenesis, translation into clinical trials has so far proved inconclusive. This chapter will not deal with preclinical studies, which have been already critically reviewed.[5–7]

Early Acute Symptomatic and Late Unprovoked Post-traumatic Seizures

In daily practice, post-traumatic epilepsy can be diagnosed by any of the following conditions: "(1) At least two unprovoked post-traumatic seizures occurring >24 hours apart; (2) one unprovoked post-traumatic seizure and a probability of further seizures similar to the general recurrence risk (at least 60%) after two unprovoked seizures, occurring over the next 10 years".[8] The electro-clinical assessment together with the imaging findings showing the TBI should "lead to a reasonable inference that the imaging abnormality is the likely cause of the patient's seizures".[3]

By definition, unprovoked post-traumatic seizures occur more than 7 days after the acute TBI.[9] They are also termed "late post-traumatic seizures" as opposed to "early post-traumatic seizures", which occur within the first 7 days after the head trauma. Although somewhat arbitrary, this straightforward temporal cut-off reflects a different underlying pathophysiology. Early post-traumatic seizures are acute symptomatic seizures occurring at the time of, or in close temporal association with, the brain injury.[9] They are due to transient and acute cellular biochemical dysfunctions leading to alterations in cortical excitability and should be regarded as a "reaction" of the brain to the lesion itself.[9] The incidence of early post-traumatic seizures ranges from 2.1% to 16.9%.[1] They carry a low risk of long-term seizure recurrence over the following 10 years (13.4% after a first seizure; 95% confidence intervals, CI = 7.0–24.8%)[10] and, hence, do not entail a diagnosis of post-traumatic epilepsy. Conversely, unprovoked seizures occurring more than 7 days after the head trauma are associated with a structural disruption of neuronal networks, increasing the excitability of the brain and leading to an enduring predisposition to generate epileptic seizures (i.e., post-traumatic epilepsy).[11] The estimated incidence of late post-traumatic seizures ranges from 1.9% to 30%.[1] A first unprovoked post-traumatic seizure has a risk of seizure recurrence over the next 10 years of 46.6% (95% CI = 30.4–66.3%).[10] Hence, the risk of long-term seizure recurrence after a first unprovoked post-traumatic seizure is significantly higher than after a first acute symptomatic post-traumatic seizure (p < 0.001).[10] However, in this study the risk of seizure recurrence over the next 10 years after a first unprovoked post-traumatic seizure was lower than the threshold of 60% required for the diagnosis of epilepsy after a single epileptic crisis,[1] and the upper confidence interval was only slightly higher. It should be noticed that this study was conducted in patients with TBI, but no details on severity or characteristics of head trauma were provided.[10] Of note, a previous longitudinal cohort study conducted in 63 patients with moderate to severe head trauma developing late post-traumatic seizures showed a cumulative incidence of recurrent late seizures of 86% by approximately 2 years.[12] Factors increasing the risk of long-term seizure recurrence should be, hence, considered on an individual basis: they include cerebral contusion and intracerebral hematoma, skull fracture, bony skull defect or penetrating injuries (e.g., bone or metal fragments, craniectomy or cranial surgery), loss of consciousness or amnesia lasting more than one day, post-traumatic seizures within the first week, severity of head trauma and age ≥ 65 years at the time of TBI.[1, 4] Adequate knowledge of these variables is important to clinically evaluate the risk of seizure recurrence and epilepsy after a single unprovoked seizure.

Epileptogenesis after Traumatic Brain Injury

In patients developing post-traumatic epilepsy there is usually a period of time of different duration, during which no epileptic seizures occur. During this clinically silent period, the brain undergoes progressive neuronal changes, which increase its excitability and eventually lead to the occurrence of recurrent spontaneous seizures or post-traumatic epilepsy.[13] This dynamic and chronic process is known as epileptogenesis and occurs in any patient developing structural epilepsy after an initial brain injury, irrespective of its etiology (e.g., stroke, tumor, trauma) (Figure 12.1).

Molecular and cellular alterations occurring in the brain after a brain-damaging insult include: selective neuronal cell death and apoptosis, changes in membrane properties, mitochondrial changes, receptor changes (e.g. loss of GABAergic receptors), deafferentation and collateral sprouting.[7, 13] These changes lead to circuitry reorganization and, hence, to permanent hyperexcitability and development of recurrent spontaneous seizures (epilepsy).[13]

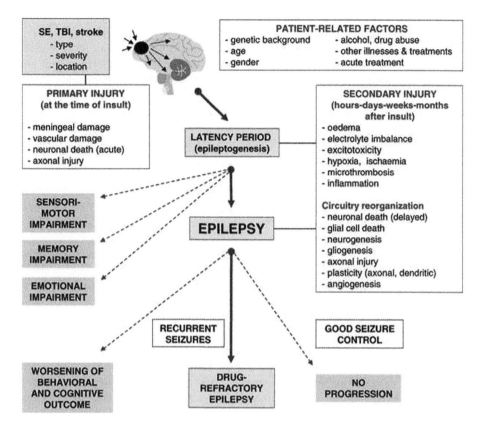

Figure 12.1 Factors influencing epileptogenesis after status epilepticus, TBI or stroke. The primary brain insult leads to "parallel and sequential molecular and cellular events that lead to various functional impairments, including sensorimotor, memory and emotional decline as well as epileptogenesis".[13] During the process of epileptogenesis, the neuronal circuitry reorganization leads to increased hyperexcitability and the occurrence of recurrent spontaneous seizures. Reproduced from Pitkänen et al (2007),[13] with permission. Blackwell Publishing, Inc. ©International League Against Epilepsy.

Recent data have shown that neuroinflammation following a TBI plays a relevant role in increasing the propensity to epileptic seizures through a variety of mechanisms, such as the activation of microglia and astrocytes, release of cytokines, disruption of the brain-blood barrier and progressive brain edema.[14] Intriguingly, a polymorphism of the interleukin-1β (IL-1β rs1143634), which is a pro-inflammatory cytokine released in the brain by astrocytes and microglia, was found to be associated with post-traumatic epilepsy in 47.7% of the cases.[15] This finding suggests that genetics may also influence the neuroinflammatory cascade and epileptogenesis after a neurotrauma.

Clinical Challenges in Antiepileptogenesis Trials

Antiepileptogenesis treatments are intended to modify the process of epileptogenesis, preventing or minimizing the risk of developing structural epilepsy after an insult to the brain. Clinical trials assessing the neuroprotective properties of compounds used to prevent epilepsy face many methodological issues. These challenges apply also to antiepileptogenesis trials of post-traumatic seizures, which are acknowledged to be more complex and expensive than conventional pharmacological studies in epilepsy.[16]

Antiepileptogenesis trials require longer duration and follow-up than trials assessing drugs for the treatment of epilepsy as seizures and epilepsy may develop even several years after the primary brain lesion.[16] More specifically, most patients (86%) with a first late post-traumatic seizures develop a second seizure within 2 years[12]; the risk remains remarkable in the following years, and it is higher following severe than moderate TBI (10 versus 30 years).[4] A long trial is, hence, needed to adequately evaluate the efficacy of the tested drug in preventing the occurrence of spontaneous seizures and structural epilepsy. It is, however, worth considering that a longer duration of the study translates into higher rates of patients lost to follow-up, which would affect the power of the study and make it less informative. At the same time, a large number of subjects recruited to compensate for the expected high proportion of patients lost to follow-up would inevitably lead to high costs. Conducting the study in an unselected population (i.e., in patients with low baseline risk of developing structural epilepsy after a brain injury) would also require the inclusion of a large number of patients to obtain informative results, again resulting in high costs.[16] Conversely, carrying out an antiepileptogenesis trial in a selected population (i.e., adopting a population enrichment design) would increase the informative value of the study and its feasibility by including a lower number of patients and reducing costs.[16–18] The identification of patient at high risk of developing post-TBI epilepsy on the basis of reliable predictors is required to design an effective antiepileptogenesis trial.[16, 19] Using a cohort from the US Traumatic Brain Injury Model Systems National Database, a model to predict the risk of post-traumatic seizures was recently developed. The model identified subdural hematoma, contusion load, craniotomy, craniectomy, early post-traumatic seizures and preinjury incarceration as predictors for post-traumatic seizures at 1 and 2 years after the injury.[20] This model showed fair to good predictive accuracy and could be used to identify and select a study population of patients at high risk of developing late post-traumatic seizures.

Other methodological issues which should be carefully considered in antiepileptogenesis studies after a neurotrauma include the co-occurrence of risk factors (e.g., severe head trauma and associated craniectomy or craniotomy), which could compete for the development of epilepsy in the target population and the need for rapid informed consent (including, whenever required and applicable, surrogate and waiver for informed consent).[16–18]

A further crucial issue is the need to disentangle the antiseizure effect of a drug from its antiepileptogenic effect. This can be achieved only if the prevention trial first assesses the antiseizure effect in a randomized controlled phase (usually versus placebo) and then the antiepileptogenic effect after washout.[18]

Other aspects to be considered concern the ascertainment of diagnosis among participants. Subclinical early post-traumatic seizures can go unnoticed, particularly in patients with impairment of consciousness or sedation.[2] Continuous video-EEG monitoring could enable to detect subclinical seizures, but this would be rather unfeasible and expensive in a large sample.[21] Furthermore, detecting late post-traumatic seizures will be even more difficult, unless patients are under close medical supervision during the entire study duration and investigators have a low threshold for suspecting seizures and asking for EEG monitoring. However, this could be hard to reach in a trial with long duration and not conducted in specialized epilepsy centers.

Finally, patients with TBI allocated to any arm should not use other agents with neuroprotective potential, in order to isolate the antiepileptogenic effect of the tested compound. If study groups receive concomitant interventions, the risk of co-intervention bias is particularly high. Unfortunately, benzodiazepines or barbiturates are frequently used for patients with severe TBI requiring sedation, and they could influence the outcome independently from the medication being studied.

Antiepileptogenic Therapies for Preventing Post-traumatic Seizures: The Evidence from the Literature

On May 28 2019, we performed a systematic search of MEDLINE (accessed through PubMed) to identify any randomized controlled trial (RCT) or systematic review assessing the use of AEDs or other neuroprotective agents for the primary prevention of post-traumatic seizures. The following search strategy was used: "(epilepsy OR seizure*) AND randomi* AND trauma".

With the aim to focus on post-traumatic seizures and provide specific data about this condition, we included only studies restricted to TBI and excluded those performed in patients undergoing brain surgery (craniectomy or craniotomy) for other indications, like brain tumors or primary intracerebral hemorrhage. Additionally, we included only RCTs and high-quality systematic reviews of the literature to rely on the highest currently available evidence.

In total, 196 results were retrieved; among them, a recent Cochrane systematic review of RCTs compared the efficacy of AEDs and neuroprotective agents with placebo, usual care or other pharmacologic agents for the prevention of post-traumatic epilepsy in people with TBI of any severity.[22] The outcomes measured included early (within 1 week of trauma) and late (later than 1 week post-trauma) seizures (Table 12.1).

No additional RCTs have been published after the aforementioned Cochrane work, which currently represents the best source of information to get guidance on the choice of antiepileptogenic therapies for preventing post-traumatic seizures. The main results are reported in the following sections.[22]

Early Acute Symptomatic Post-traumatic Seizures

The Cochrane review included five trials (987 participants), which compared either phenytoin (PHT) or carbamazepine (CBZ) with placebo or usual care in children to adults and provided data on the occurrence of early acute symptomatic post-traumatic seizures.[23–27] The quantitative synthesis of the results favored the use of AEDs compared with the control group (occurrence in treatment group 25/499, 5.0% versus 68/488, 13.9%; risk ratio [RR] 0.42; 95% confidence interval [CI] 0.23–0.73). The overall quality of evidence was judged to be low due to serious risk of selective reporting bias and imprecision of results.

A further study compared magnesium sulfate with placebo in 499 participants.[28] Only 1 of 250 patients (0.4%) in the magnesium group had an early post-traumatic seizure, compared to none (0/249) in the placebo group (RR 2.99; 95% CI 0.12–73.00). Both groups were treated with PHT for the first week after the head trauma, and this may have contributed to the very low seizure rate. The overall quality of evidence was judged to be low due to serious risk of bias and imprecision of results.

One study compared PHT to valproic acid (VPA),[29] and another compared PHT to levetiracetam (LEV).[30] Both studies failed to find statistically meaningful differences between PHT and the active comparators (2/132 in the PHT group versus 11/247 in the

Table 12.1 Characteristics of included studies

Study	World region/Country	Interventions	Age	Severity of head trauma	Number of participants	Duration of treatment	Duration of follow-up	Occurrence of early acute symptomatic post-traumatic seizures	Occurrence of late unprovoked post-traumatic seizures	Notes
Antiepileptic drug versus placebo or current standard of care										
Glotzner et al, 1983[23]	Europe	Carbamazepine (dose according to serum levels 300–600 µg) versus placebo	>15 years	Moderate and severe	Carbamazepine: 75 Placebo: 76	18–24 months	18–24 months	8/75 versus 22/76	14/75 versus 20/76	Seizures identified clinically and with EEG Intervention started immediately after trauma Most patients received phenobarbital, diazepam or both in the first week as treatment of brain edema
McQueen et al, 1983[31]	Europe	Phenytoin (dose adjusted to achieve serum levels 40–80 µmol/L) versus placebo	5–65 years	Not specified	Phenytoin: 84 Placebo: 80	12 months	2 years		8/84 versus 7/80	Seizures identified clinically Intervention started before post-traumatic seizures (not further details)
Young et al, 1983[24]	USA	Phenytoin (initial dose 11 mg/kg plus 13 mg/kg intramuscularly, then 8.8 mg/kg/day) versus placebo	All ages	Severe	Phenytoin: 136 Placebo: 108	7 days (short-term) and 18 months (long-term)	1 week to 18 months	5/136 versus 4/108	13/105 versus 8/74 1.15	Not specified how seizures were identified
Temkin et al, 1990[25]	USA	Phenytoin (loading dose: 20 mg/kg, then dose adjusted to achieve serum levels 40–80 µmol/L) versus	34±18 years	Severe	Phenytoin: 208 Placebo: 196	12 months	2 years	7/208 versus 26/196	36/170 versus 26/153	Seizures identified clinically Intervention started within 24 hours of trauma

Study	World region/Country	Interventions	Age	Severity of head trauma	Number of participants	Duration of treatment	Duration of follow-up	Occurrence of early acute symptomatic post-traumatic seizures	Occurrence of late unprovoked post-traumatic seizures	Notes
Pechadre et al., 1991[26]	Europe	Phenytoin (10 mg/kg at 40 mg/min) versus placebo	5–60 years	Severe	Phenytoin: 34 Placebo: 52	3 months and 1 year	2 years	2/34 versus 13/52	2/34 versus 22/52	Intervention started within 24 hours of trauma
Manaka et al., 1992[32]	Japan	Phenobarbital 10–25 µg/mL, started 4 weeks after head trauma versus usual standard of care	7–88 years	Not specified	Phenobarbital: 50 Usual care: 76	2 years	5 years		8/50 versus 8/76	Not specified how seizures were identified Phenobarbital started 4 weeks after trauma Not specified how many patients with usual care treatment received antiepileptic drugs
Young et al., 2004[27]	USA	Phenytoin (loading dose 18 mg/kg, then maintenance 2 mg/kg every 8 hours) versus placebo	<10 years	Moderate to severe	Phenytoin: 47 Placebo: 56	5 days	30 days	3/46 versus 3/56		Seizures identified clinically and with EEG Intervention started before post-traumatic seizures (not further details)
Other neuroprotective agents versus placebo										
Temkin et al., 2007[28]	USA	Magnesium sulfate (high dose 1.2–2.5 mmol/L; low dose: 1.0–1.85 mmol/L) versus placebo	>14 years	Moderate or severe	Magnesium sulfate high dose: 59 Magnesium sulfate low dose: 191 Placebo: 249	5 days	6 months	1/250 versus 0/249	15/249 versus 14/249	Not specified how seizures were identified Not specified when interventions were given

Table 12.1 (Cont.)

Study	World region/Country	Interventions	Age	Severity of head trauma	Number of participants	Duration of treatment	Duration of follow-up	Occurrence of early acute symptomatic post-traumatic seizures	Occurrence of late unprovoked post-traumatic seizures	Notes
Antiepileptic drugs compared to other antiepileptic drugs										
Temkin et al, 1999[29]	USA	Phenytoin 1 week (loading dose: 20 mg/kg, then 5 mg/kg/day) versus valproate 1 and 6 months (loading dose: 20 mg/kg, then 15 mg/kg/day)	Phenytoin 1 week: 36±16 years Valproate 1 month: 40±19 years Valproate 6 months: 36±16 years	Severe	Phenytoin 1 week: 132 Valproate 1 month: 120 Valproate 6 months: 127	1 week, 1 month, 6 months	2 years	2/132 versus 11/247	17/123 versus 39/221	Seizures identified clinically
Szaflarski et al, 2010[30]	USA	Phenytoin (loading dose: 20 mg/kg, then maintenance: 5 mg/kg/day) versus levetiracetam (loading dose: 20 mg, then maintenance 1000 mg every 12 hours)	17–80 years	Severe or subarachnoid hemorrhage	Phenytoin: 18 Levetiracetam: 34	7 days	3 and 6 months	3/18 versus 5/34	0/14 versus 1/20	Seizures identified clinically and with EEG Not specified when interventions were given

VPA group; RR 0.34; 95% CI 0.08–1.51[29]; 3/18 in the PHT group versus 5/34 in the LEV group; RR 1.13; 95% CI 0.31–4.21[30]).

Late Unprovoked Post-traumatic Seizures

Six trials (1,029 participants) were included in the Cochrane review.[23–26, 31,32] One study compared phenobarbital with usual care,[32] one compared CBZ with placebo,[23] and the remaining four PHT with placebo.[24–26, 31] The pooled results did not show statistically significant differences between AEDs and placebo or usual care (occurrence in treatment group: 81/518, 15.6% versus 91/511, 17.8%; RR 0.91, 95% CI 0.57–1.467); the overall quality of evidence was judged to be very low due to serious risk of bias, inconsistency and imprecision of results.

A further study compared magnesium sulfate with placebo in 499 participants.[28] No difference was found in the occurrence of unprovoked post-traumatic seizures between patients allocated to magnesium sulfate (15/250, 6%) and those receiving placebo (14/249, 5.6%) (RR 1.07; 95% CI 0.53–2.17). Of note, both groups were treated with PHT for the first week after the head trauma.

One study compared PHT to VPA,[29] and another PHT to LEV.[30] Both studies failed to find statistical differences between PHT and the active comparator (17/123 in the PHT group versus 39/221 in the VPA group; RR 0.78; 95% CI 0.46–1.32[29]; 0/14 in the PHT group versus 1/20 in the LEV group; RR 0.47; 95% CI 0.02–10.69[30]). Although the RCT comparing PHT to LEV found a significant improvement in the Extended Glasgow Outcome Scale with lower disability at 6 months in patients receiving LEV,[30] no difference in the occurrence of late post-traumatic seizure was found between the groups.

Results of the study comparing PHT to LEV were included in two subsequent systematic reviews of the literature.[21, 33] which failed to find other RCTs with the same comparators and provided the same conclusions of the Cochrane analysis.

Adverse Events

Only two RCTs, both comparing PHT to placebo, reported adverse events,[25, 31] No statistical difference was found between the groups with regard to the occurrence of any serious event (42/292, 14.4% in the PHT group versus 26/276, 9.5% in the placebo group; RR 1.65, 95% CI 0.73–3.66); the overall quality of evidence was judged to be low due to serious risk of selection bias and imprecision of results.

The same two studies reported the occurrence of skin rashes, failing to show a difference between PHT and placebo (30/292, 10.3% in the PHT group versus 18/276, 6.5% in the placebo group; RR 1.65 99% CI 0.54–5.04; 568 participants); the overall quality of evidence was judged to be low due to serious risk of bias and imprecision of results.

Implications for Clinical Practice

A comprehensive review of the available literature has shown that the prophylactic use of AEDs is effective in reducing the risk of developing early (acute symptomatic) post-traumatic seizures compared to placebo or usual care in patients with severe TBI. The overall evidence was, however, graded to be of low-quality due to the risk of biases in included studies and imprecision of estimates. The latter is likely attributable to the small number of participants included in each trial.

Considering that early post-traumatic seizures carry a low risk of long-term seizure recurrence (i.e., post-traumatic epilepsy),[10] the use of AEDs should be restricted to the acute phase (7 days) and not prolonged beyond that.[34–36] In other words, patients with TBI do not generally require long-term AED treatment since their risk of developing post-traumatic epilepsy is low. The acute antiepileptic treatment to decrease the incidence of early post-traumatic seizures should be taken into consideration "when the overall benefit is thought to outweigh the complications associated with such treatment. However, early post traumatic seizures have not been associated with worse outcomes".[36]

With regards to the choice of AED, the available evidence supports the use of PHT, starting with an intravenous loading dose initiated as soon as possible after severe TBI.[35] The use of PHT appears also to be a cost-effective option compared to LEV,[37] without difference in terms of occurrence of early post-traumatic seizures, adverse events or mortality,[38] Several issues should be, however, carefully considered when choosing PHT. It is associated with dermatological adverse events and induces cytochrome P450 enzymes, leading to drug–drug interactions.[39] Furthermore, PHT has a nonlinear pharmacokinetics and a narrow therapeutic index, requiring frequent serum concentration, especially because of the alterations in its metabolism occurring after severe neurotrauma.[40–42] The availability of generic LEV may change the pharmacoeconomic scenario. Indeed, LEV is increasingly used in primary prevention of early post-traumatic seizures due to its ease of use, favorable safety profile and lack of pharmacokinetic interactions.[43] In a US survey, most epilepsy specialists (74%) considered LEV to be the drug of choice for this indication compared to only 10% preferring PHT.[44] Conversely, a survey of UK neurosurgical use of AEDs in acute TBI showed that among physicians prescribing drugs for acute seizure prophylaxis 65.6% chose PHT and 21.9% LEV.[21] These figures emphasize the need for an adequately powered non-inferiority RCT to determine whether there is equipoise between these two drugs. [21]

So far, there is a lack of evidence to support the use of other neuroprotective agents for the primary prevention of early post-traumatic seizures.

Relying on the available evidence, it is hard to make recommendations for the long-term use of AEDs to prevent post-traumatic epilepsy. The lack of difference between AEDs and placebo in the occurrence of late post-traumatic seizures could be attributed to the small sample size and insufficient statistical power to detect a difference between the arms. Hence, high-quality and adequately powered trials conducted in a selected population at high risk of developing late post-traumatic seizures are required to draw definite conclusions on the effectiveness of long-term prophylactic treatment.

Further studies to explore the antiepileptogenic and neuroprotective effects of anti-inflammatory and immune-modulatory therapies should be also warranted.

References

1. Frey LC. Epidemiology of posttraumatic epilepsy: a critical review. *Epilepsia* 2003;44:11–17.

2. Agrawal A, Timothy J, Pandit L, Manju M. Post-traumatic epilepsy: an overview. *Clin Neurol Neurosurg* 2006;108:433–9.

3. Scheffer IE, Berkovic S, Capovilla G, et al. ILAE classification of the epilepsies: Position paper of the ILAE Commission for Classification and Terminology. *Epilepsia* 2017;58:512–21.

4. Annegers JF, Hauser WA, Coan SP, Rocca WA. A population-based study of

seizures after traumatic brain injuries. *N Engl J Med* 1998;338:20–4.

5. Pitkänen A, McIntosh TK. Animal models of post-traumatic epilepsy. *J Neurotrauma* 2006;23:241–61

6. Pitkänen A, Bolkvadze T, Immonen R. Anti-epileptogenesis in rodent post-traumatic epilepsy models. *Neurosci Lett* 2011;497:163–71.

7. Pitkänen A, Immonen R. Epilepsy related to traumatic brain injury. *Neurotherapeutics* 2014;11:286–96.

8. Fisher RS, Acevedo C, Arzimanoglou A, et al. ILAE official report: a practical clinical definition of epilepsy. *Epilepsia* 2014;55:475–82.

9. Beghi E, Carpio A, Forsgren L, et al. Recommendation for a definition of acute symptomatic seizure. *Epilepsia* 2010;51:671–5.

10. Hesdorffer DC, Benn EK, Cascino GD, Hauser WA. Is a first acute symptomatic seizure epilepsy? Mortality and risk for recurrent seizure. *Epilepsia* 2009;50:1102–8.

11. Fisher RS, van Emde Boas W, et al. Epileptic seizures and epilepsy: definitions proposed by the International League Against Epilepsy (ILAE) and the International Bureau for Epilepsy (IBE). *Epilepsia* 2005;46:470–2.

12. Haltiner AM, Temkin NR, Dikmen SS. Risk of seizure recurrence after the first late posttraumatic seizure. *Arch Phys Med Rehabil* 1997;78:835–40.

13. Pitkänen A, Kharatishvili I, Karhunen H, et al. Epileptogenesis in experimental models. *Epilepsia* 2007;48:13–20

14. Webster KM, Sun M, Crack P, O'Brien TJ, Shultz SR, Semple BD. Inflammation in epileptogenesis after traumatic brain injury. *J Neuroinflammation* 2017;14:10.

15. Cotter D, Kelso A, Neligan A. Genetic biomarkers of posttraumatic epilepsy: A systematic review. *Seizure* 2017;46:53–8.

16. Trinka E, Brigo F. Antiepileptogenesis in humans: disappointing clinical evidence and ways to move forward. *Curr Opin Neurol* 2014;27:227–35.

17. Mani R, Pollard J, Dichter MA. Human clinical trials in antiepileptogenesis. *Neurosci Lett* 2011; 497:251–6.

18. Schmidt D. Is antiepileptogenesis a realistic goal in clinical trials? Concerns and new horizons. *Epileptic Disord* 2012;14:105–13.

19. Engel J Jr, Pitkänen A, Loeb JA, et al. Epilepsy biomarkers. *Epilepsia* 2013;54:61–9.

20. Ritter AC, Wagner AK, Szaflarski JP, et al. Prognostic models for predicting posttraumatic seizures during acute hospitalization, and at 1 and 2 years following traumatic brain injury. *Epilepsia* 2016;57:1503–14.

21. Bakr A, Belli A. A systematic review of levetiracetam versus phenytoin in the prevention of late post-traumatic seizures and survey of UK neurosurgical prescribing practice of antiepileptic medication in acute traumatic brain injury. *Br J Neurosurg* 2018;32:237–44.

22. Thompson K, Pohlmann-Eden B, Campbell LA, Abel H. Pharmacological treatments for preventing epilepsy following traumatic head injury. *Cochrane Database Syst Rev*. 2015;CD009900.

23. Glotzner FL, Haubitz I, Miltner F, Kapp G, Pflughaupt KW. Seizure prevention using carbamazepine following severe brain injuries [Anfallsprophylaxe mit Carbamazepin nach schweren Schadelhirnverletzungen *Neurochirurgia* 1983;26:66–79.

24. Young B, Rapp RP, Norton JA, Haack D, Tibbs PA, Bean JR. Failure of prophylactically administered phenytoin to prevent late posttraumatic seizures. *J Neurosurg* 1983;58:236–41.

25. Temkin NR, Dikmen SS, Wilensky AJ, Keihm J, Chabal S, Winn HR. A randomized double-blind study of phenytoin for the prevention of post-traumatic seizures. *N Eng J Med* 1990;323:497–502.

26. Pechadre JC, Lauxerois M, Colnet G, et al. Prevention of late posttraumatic epilepsy by phenytoin in severe brain injuries, 2 years' follow-up [Prevention de l'epilepsie post–traumatique tardive par phenytoine

dans les traumatismes crannies graves, suivi durant 2 ans *Presse Medicale* 1991;20:841–5.

27. Young KD, Okada PJ, Sokolove PE, et al. A randomized, double-blinded, placebo-controlled trial of phenytoin for the prevention of early posttraumatic seizures in children with moderate to severe blunt head injury. *Ann Emerg Med* 2004;43:435–46.

28. Temkin NR, Anderson GC, Winn HR, et al. Magnesium sulfate for neuroprotection after traumatic brain injury: a randomized controlled trial. *Lancet Neurol* 2007;6:29–38.

29. Temkin NR, Dikmen SS, Anderson GD, et al. Valproate therapy for prevention of posttraumatic seizures: a randomized trial. *J Neurosurg* 1999;91:593–600.

30. Szaflarski JP, Sangha KS, Lindsell CJ, Shutter LA. Prospective, randomized, single-blinded comparative trial of intravenous levetiracetam versus phenytoin for seizure prophylaxis. *Neurocrit Care* 2010;12:165–72.

31. McQueen JK, Blackwood DHR, Harris P, Kalbag RM, Johnson AL. Low risk of late post-traumatic seizures following severe head injury: implications for clinical trials of prophylaxis. *J Neurol Neurosurg Psychiatr* 1983;46:899–904.

32. Manaka S. Cooperative prospective study on posttraumatic epilepsy: risk factors and the effect of prophylactic anticonvulsant. *Japan J Psychiatr Neurol* 1992;46:311–5.

33. Yang Y, Zheng F, Xu X, Wang X. Levetiracetam versus phenytoin for seizure prophylaxis following traumatic brain injury: A systematic review and meta-analysis. *CNS Drugs.* 2016;30:677–88.

34. Beghi E. Overview of studies to prevent posttraumatic epilepsy. *Epilepsia* 2003;44:21–6.

35. Chang BS, Lowenstein DH. Quality Standards Subcommittee of the American Academy of Neurology. Practice parameter: antiepileptic drug prophylaxis in severe traumatic brain injury: report of the Quality Standards Subcommittee of the American Academy of Neurology. *Neurology* 2003; 60:10–16.

36. Carney N, Totten AM, O'Reilly C, et al. Guidelines for the Management of Severe Traumatic Brain Injury, Fourth Edition. *Neurosurgery.* 2017;80:6–15.

37. Cotton BA, Kao LS, Kozar R, Holcomb JB. Cost-utility analysis of levetiracetam and phenytoin for posttraumatic seizure prophylaxis. *J Trauma* 2011;71:375–9.

38. Inaba K, Menaker J, Branco BC, et al. A prospective multicenter comparison of levetiracetam versus phenytoin for early posttraumatic seizure prophylaxis. *J Trauma Acute Care Surg.* 2013;74:766–71

39. Zaccara G, Perucca E. Interactions between antiepileptic drugs, and between antiepileptic drugs and other drugs. *Epileptic Disord* 2014;16:409–31.

40. Shohrati M, Rouini MR, Mojtahedzadeh M, Firouzabadi M. Evaluation of phenytoin pharmacokinetics in neurotrauma patients. *Daru* 2007;15:34–40.

41. Sadeghi K, Hadi F, Ahmadi A, et al. Total phenytoin concentration is not well correlated with active free drug in critically-ill head trauma patients. *J Res Pharm Pract* 2013;2:105–9

42. Alimardani S, Sadrai S, Masoumi HT, et al. Pharmacokinetic behavior of phenytoin in head trauma and cerebrovascular accident patients in an Iranian population. *J Res Pharm Pract.* 2017;6:217–22.

43. Kruer RM, Harris LH, Goodwin H, et al. Changing trends in the use of seizure prophylaxis after traumatic brain injury: a shift from phenytoin to levetiracetam. *J Crit Care* 2013;28:883.e9–13

44. Szaflarski JP. Is there equipoise between phenytoin and levetiracetam for seizure prevention in traumatic brain injury? *Epilepsy Curr* 2015;15:94–7.

Chapter 13

Effects of Antiepileptic Drugs on Cognition

Kimford Meador and Zahra Sadat-Hossieny

Introduction

Traumatic brain injury (TBI) can result in cognitive and behavioral deficits as well as seizures. Anti-seizure medications (ASMs) are the mainstay of therapy for seizure management. Thus, the effects of ASMs on cognition are vital to the practice of any healthcare provider who provides treatment for patients with TBI and seizures. ASMs exert their effects on cognition through modulating the different modalities of cognitive processing and also through affecting behavior and psychology. The most common effects of ASMs on cognitive functions include reductions in psychomotor speed, attention (particularly sustained or complex attention), dual processing, memory and naming or word finding.[1] ASMs can affect behavior by producing positive effects such as mood stabilization, or by producing adverse effects such as depression, irritability, agitation or psychosis.

Selecting the appropriate ASM for each patient can be done by weighing the positive and negative cognitive effects of each medication. Research has shown that benzodiazepines, phenobarbital and topiramate have higher associations with adverse cognitive effects compared to other ASMs. Positive behavioral modulation has been shown with carbamazepine, lamotrigine and valproate while negative behavioral and mood effects have been seen with levetiracetam, phenobarbital and topiramate. Further attention must be given to therapeutic ranges of drugs, blood levels, rates of drug titration, polypharmacy and the age of the patient. Higher doses and higher blood levels may result in more cognitive side effects. There is an increased risk of cognitive side effects when ASMs are up titrated quickly, and insufficient time is given in the first few weeks for habituation. Decreasing the number of ASMs may improve cognition and even decrease seizures. The elderly have increased vulnerability to the cognitive side effects of medications.[1] The most favorable outcomes are reached when medications are selected with the specific patient and their cognitive reserve in mind. The following sections will examine research related to many ASMs and their effects on cognition.

Carbamazepine, Phenobarbital, Phenytoin and Valproate

Carbamazepine and phenytoin have similar mechanisms of action, preventing repetitive and sustained firing of neurons via action on voltage-gated sodium channels. In addition, they also share similar cognitive side effect profiles. They were compared in a double-blind, randomized, crossover, monotherapy design study that controlled for anticonvulsant blood levels, and the results showed that there is no difference in the cognitive effects of the two medications.[2, 3] The only significant differences found in this study included decreased performance on the finger tapping test for phenytoin in comparison to carbamazepine and decreased performance on the Stroop test for carbamazepine in comparison with phenytoin. Both valproate and phenobarbital have multiple mechanisms of action, but both exert effects by making the inhibitory neurotransmitter GABA either more available or more effective. Valproate also blocks voltage-gated sodium channels, and phenobarbital also causes decreased efficacy of the excitatory neurotransmitter glutamate. Phenobarbital was found to have worse cognitive effects than both phenytoin and carbamazepine.[2] A placebo-controlled, prospective, randomized, double-blind, parallel group study of anticonvulsant withdrawal in a patient population taking a single ASM with completely controlled seizures found improved cognitive function on neuropsychiatric tests once the ASM was withdrawn compared to patients in whom ASM was not withdrawn.[4] It is important to note that being on any of these ASMs, when compared to being on no ASMs, resulted in significantly poorer performance on a battery of neuropsychiatric tests (performance was worse in 52% of tested variables).

Brivaracetam

Brivaracetam was approved for clinical use in patients with focal onset seizures in February 2016 and is among the newest ASMs. It is an analog of levetiracetam and has highly selective binding for a novel brain-specific binding site synaptic vesicle protein 2A (SV2A).[5] A randomized, double-blind, placebo-controlled, four-way crossover design study in healthy volunteers comparing acute single doses of brivaracetam, levetiracetam, lorazepam and placebo found no significant difference in cognitive testing between placebo, levetiracetam and brivaracetam; however, it did find a significant decline in cognitive tasks with lorazepam.[6] In a study of brivaracetam, 36 patients who were suffering from adverse side effects of levetiracetam were switched to brivaracetam: 24 of these patients (66.67%) experienced a clinically meaningful reduction in side effects after the switch.[7] Brivaracetam was discontinued in 26/93 patients (28%). In the ten who switched back to levetiracetam, seven had a reduction in adverse effects. However, no randomized, double-blind comparisons of brivaracetam and levetiracetam behavioral effects have been conducted.

Eslicarbazepine

Eslicarbazepine is a new generation ASM chemically related to carbamazepine and oxcarbazepine but has structural and metabolic differences. In a randomized, double-blind, crossover design comparing eslicarbazepine with immediate-release carbamazepine in healthy volunteers, eslicarbazepine demonstrated fewer adverse neuropsychological effects than carbamazepine.[8]

Gabapentin

Gabapentin was approved by the FDA in 1993 as an adjuvant for treatment of focal onset seizures. Studies examining the cognitive effects of gabapentin have found few cognitive side effects from gabapentin when used in the treatment of epilepsy. The effect of gabapentin on cognition was assessed at doses of 1,200 mg, 1,800 mg and 2,400 mg per day in a double-blind, placebo-controlled, add-on crossover study and reported no substantial effect on composite psychomotor/memory scores, nor any alteration in any self-assessment subscore.[9] A direct comparison of gabapentin, carbamazepine and placebo in a double-blind, randomized, crossover study of healthy volunteers found significantly better performance with gabapentin than carbamazepine on 26% of variables in cognitive tests.[10] A randomized, double-blind, parallel group study of carbamazepine and gabapentin in healthy volunteers found both ASMs caused EEG slowing and worsening function on cognitive testing but with no significant difference between the two drugs.[11]

Lacosamide

Lacosamide was approved in 2008 by the FDA for adjunctive treatment of focal onset seizures. Unlike other sodium channel ASMs, lacosamide enhances the slow inactivation of voltage-gated sodium channels without affecting their fast inactivation. The effects of lacosamide and carbamazepine were compared in a randomized, double-blind, crossover study in healthy subjects, which found that carbamazepine had worse scores than lacosamide for the primary composite neuropsychological outcome and for the composite EEG score. Lacosamide was better than carbamazepine on 36% of the neuropsychological tests.[12]

Lamotrigine

Lamotrigine was approved for the treatment of epilepsy in 1994 and acts on the voltage gated sodium channels. Since its approval, there have been many studies that show a superior cognitive profile for lamotrigine in comparison to other ASMs including topiramate, phenytoin, carbamazepine and diazepam.[13-18] When compared to carbamazepine, patients on lamotrigine performed better on 19/40 (48%) variables in cognitive tests.[13] Direct comparison of lamotrigine to topiramate in healthy volunteers yielded better performance for patients on lamotrigine in 33/41 (80%) variables without adjustment for drug levels and 19/41 (46%) with adjustment for drug levels.[14] Lamotrigine was compared to valproate and placebo in healthy adults, and results showed that patients on lamotrigine performed better compared to placebo on three of four tests of reaction time. Patients on lamotrigine performed better compared to valproate on two of four tests of reaction time and had significant reduction in drug-related cognitive complaints. Patients on lamotrigine had improvement in five of six mood scales while patients on valproate had worsening on four of six mood scales in the same study.[15] A separate study found significant unsteadiness in patients given phenytoin, drowsiness in patients given diazepam and found no significant side effects in patients taking lamotrigine.[16] Lamotrigine's preferable cognitive profile as well as its effectiveness as an ASM and a mood stabilizer is often of great benefit in epilepsy patients who frequently require management of mood and cognition in addition to seizure control.[19]

Levetiracetam

Levetiracetam was approved by the FDA for the treatment of epilepsy in 1999. The mechanism by which it exerts its antiseizure properties are not completely understood, but it binds to SV2A, a synaptic vesicle glycoprotein, inhibits presynaptic calcium channels and reduces neurotransmitter release. Levetiracetam is often a first choice in the treatment of epilepsy due to its lack of interaction with other medications and its favorable cognitive profile. The cognitive effects of levetiracetam in comparison to carbamazepine were compared in a randomized, double-blind, two-period crossover design study[19] – the study found that levetiracetam had significantly fewer cognitive effects on 44% of tested variables. This data, when considered in combination with studies comparing carbamazepine to older ASMs like phenytoin, phenobarbital and valproate, indicates that levetiracetam also has fewer cognitive side effects than the listed older ASMs. Although the cognitive profile of levetiracetam is favorable, it may lead to unfavorable psychiatric side effects in the form of worsening depression, irritation or agitation. For example, the behavioral complications of levetiracetam in comparison to gabapentin and lamotrigine have been evaluated, and it has become apparent that levetiracetam carries a higher negative behavioral side effect profile.[20–21] Pyridoxine has been examined as an add-on treatment to decrease the behavioral side effects of levetiracetam. A randomized, single-blind, case-control trial in children looked at the effect of adding pyridoxine for patients who had been taking levetiracetam for 1 month and were experiencing negative side effects. The study found that 92% of patients who initiated pyridoxine after 1 month of LEV treatment did not need to change or suspend levetiracetam, and behavioral adverse effects of levetiracetam improved after 6–12 days of treatment.[22] This study supports prior case reports, but an additional randomized double-blind investigation is needed.

Oxcarbazepine

Oxcarbazepine is a structural derivative of carbamazepine and was formulated to decrease the side effect profile of carbamazepine. An open-label, randomized, active-control, three-arm, parallel-group, 6-month study compared the cognitive side effects of oxcarbazepine to carbamazepine and valproate in patients 6 to <17 years of age and disclosed no significant difference.[23] The cognitive effects of oxcarbazpine have been compared to phenytoin in adult patients with epilepsy[24] and in healthy subjects,[25] and no significant difference has been found.

Perampanel

Perampanel was approved in 2012 and works as a non-competitive antagonist of AMPA receptors. It carries a black box warning for serious psychiatric and behavioral changes such as aggression, hostility and homicidal ideation. A total of 133 patients with poorly controlled focal onset seizures were randomized to perampanel or placebo in a randomized, double-blind, placebo-controlled, adjunctive study and the cognitive effects of perampanel were evaluated.[26] No difference from placebo was seen for perampanel for global cognitive score, two of five subdomains and four other cognitive measures. Patients on perampanel performed worse than placebo in two domains: continuity of attention and speed of memory.[26] Similar results were found in a long-term, open-label follow up study on 112 patients aged 12–18.[27] This study followed patients for up to 52 weeks and found no significant cognitive effects for cognitive drug research system global cognition score, continuity of attention, quality of episodic memory, quality of working memory or speed of memory, but did find a significant decline in power of attention at end of treatment compared with baseline.[27]

Rufinamide

Rufinamide was approved for use in seizures related to Lennox–Gastaut syndrome in 2008 and is used in treatment of focal onset seizures. It is thought act through limiting the frequency of sodium dependent neuronal action potentials. A multicenter, multinational double-blind, randomized, placebo-controlled, parallel-study looked at the cognitive effects of rufinamide when given as an add-on medication for patients with poorly controlled seizures.[28] Four doses of rufinamide were administered (200 mg/day, 400 mg/day, 800 mg/day and 1,600 mg/day), and cognitive testing was performed before start of rufinamide and after 3 months of treatment. Cognitive functions (psychomotor speed and alertness, mental information processing speed and attention and working memory) showed no significant difference before and after treatment with rufinamide.

Tiagibine

Tiagabine was approved for use in epilepsy in 1998 by the FDA and works by blocking the uptake of GABA and thus reducing excitation and likelihood of seizures. Its effects on cognition were examined in a double-blind, add-on, placebo-controlled, parallel, multi-center, dose-response efficacy study in patients with focal epilepsy whose complex partial seizures were difficult to control. A total of 162 patients were randomized to placebo or tiagibine 16 mg/day, 32 mg/day or 56 mg/day. Their performance on eight cognitive tests and three measures of mood and adjustment showed no significant difference before initiation of tiagabine compared to post 12 weeks of treatment.[29]

Topiramate

Topiramate has been approved for use in the treatment of seizures since 1996. It has been shown to produce state-dependent blocking of sodium channels, enhance GABA transmission, reduce action of excitatory neurotransmitters via kainate and AMPA receptors and decrease the action of carbonic anhydrase. Patients report cognitive side effects such as speech problems or problems with word finding, psychomotor slowing and memory impairment.[30-33] These effects are more common with higher doses or rapid up titration. A multicenter, randomized, observer-blind trial looked at the cognitive effects of topiramate in comparison to valproate when added on to carbamazepine for treatment of seizures. It found a statistically significant worsening in short-term verbal memory with topiramate in comparison to valproate and placebo. This study also found that gradual introduction of topiramate (introduced at 25 mg and increased with weekly 25 mg/d increments) can decrease the extent of cognitive impairment compared to rapid introduction at higher doses (100–200 mg/day introductory dose).[34] A similar study found that patients taking topiramate performed worse than those taking valproate on two cognitive tests: the Symbol Digit Modalities Test and the Controlled Oral Word Association Test.[35] The cognitive effects of topiramate and gabapentin were compared in a double-blind, placebo-controlled study of healthy volunteers and showed that patients taking topiramate performed worse than those taking gabapentin on 12 of 24 cognitive measures.[36] The cognitive effects of topiramate were compared to lamotrigine in healthy volunteers[14] and in patients with epilepsy,[18] and significantly greater cognitive impairment was seen on multiple measures in subjects taking topiramate in both studies. The dose-dependent effects of topiramate were studied in a double-blind, placebo-controlled study on cognitively normal adults and showed that a greater number of subjects developed cognitive impairment at higher doses of topiramate, especially at doses >200 mg/day.[37]

Vigabatrin

Vigabatrin was approved for use in 2009 and works by irreversibly inhibiting the breakdown of GABA. Severe behavioral disturbances such as depression and psychosis have been reported in 3.4% of adult patients and 6% of pediatric patients started on Vigabatrin.[38] The effects of vigabatrin on cognition and quality of life were examined in patients with epilepsy in a dose-dependent fashion, and little impact was seen in cognition or quality of life with placebo versus 1 g, 3 g or 6g of Vigabatrin.[39] A separate study randomized 45 patients to vigabatrin or placebo for a double-blinded period of 20 weeks and then followed them for an 18-month open label period. Patients on vigabatrin had a significant reduction in a measure of motor speed and overall score on a design learning test in the first 20 weeks of treatment. Of the patients who continued follow-up in the open label phase, these side effects either stayed the same with treatment (did not worsen) or improved.[40]

Zonisamide

Zonisamide was approved for use in 2000 and has a mechanism of action and side effect profile that is similar to topiramate, but formal cognitive studies are inadequate and there are no head-to-head comparisons to other ASMs. A preliminary study of zonisamide and cognition found that it impaired acquisition and consolidation of new information as well as verbal learning.[41] The long-term cognitive and mood effects of zonisamide were investigated in a prospective, randomized, open-label trial in patients with epilepsy. Cognitive and mood testing was done at the beginning of the study and after 1 year of treatment and showed that zonisamide resulted in negative effects on delayed word recall, the Trail Making Test part B and verbal fluency. Worse cognitive effects were also associated with higher doses of medication.[42]

Epilepsy Surgery

Epilepsy surgery is the most effective treatment for focal epilepsy and results in seizure freedom in 58% of patients.[43] Gliotic or dysfunctional tissue is removed, thus, global cognitive decline typically does not occur and improvement in cognitive function is possible. Verbal memory decline is reported in 22% to 63% of patients who undergo left anterior temporal lobe resection, and visual memory impairments are reported in 6% to 32% of patients who undergo right anterior temporal lobe resection.[44] Cognitive side effects after resection depend on multiple variables including location of resection, functional status of the tissue being resected, age at onset of seizures, patient demographics and baseline cognitive abilities. Ancillary testing such as neuropsychiatric evaluation, fMRI and Wada testing can assist in predicting the extent of cognitive decline after surgery.[45]

Neurostimulation

Neurostimulation is being used increasingly to treat medically refractory epilepsy. The most commonly used forms of neurostimulation are vagal nerve stimulation (VNS), deep brain stimulation (DBS) and responsive neurostimulation (RNS). At 1 year, greater than 50% seizure reduction has been reported in 34% of patients with VNS, 43% of patients with DBS and 44% of patients with RNS. At 5 years, greater than 55% seizure reduction has been reported in 64% of patients with VNS, 68% of patients with DBS and 61% of patients with RNS.[45] The effects of VNS on memory are unclear, with some studies reporting improved cognitive function and some studies reporting no significant change in cognitive function. VNS has generally been associated with improvement in mood. DBS of the anterior nucleus of the thalamus has shown no objective, long-term effects on cognition or behavior. RNS has shown no cognitive side effects and even demonstrated modest improvement in verbal memory in patients with mesial temporal seizures and modest improvement in naming in patients with neocortical location of seizures. RNS has also shown significant improvements in mood at 2 years.[45-48]

Methylphenidate

The typical approach to improving the neuropsychological status of patients with epilepsy is to reduce seizures, use ASMs with fewer cognitive side effects and treat mood disorders. Direct treatment of cognitive impairments is unusual except for occasional application of cognitive behavioral therapy. Methylphenidate has been studied for treatment of cognitive impairment in epilepsy patients in a double-blind, placebo-controlled study.[49] Patients were randomized to placebo, methylphenidate 10 mg daily or methylphenidate 20 mg daily. Cognitive testing before and after treatment with methylphenidate showed statistically significant improvement in performance with both 10 mg and 20 mg doses,[49] which was maintained in a 1 month follow-up.[50] No seizures occurred as a side effect of methylphenidate use. Patients with TBI frequently suffer from acquired attentional deficit disorder, which may benefit from sympathometic treatment. However, concerns for seizure risk due to sympathometics have been raised. However, the small study in patients with epilepsy[50] and several large studies in children with attentional deficit disorder[51-52] do not reveal a risk of seizures when sympathometics are used in therapeutic dosages for attentional deficit disorder. Although additional studies are needed, methylphenidate should be considered to improve cognitive abilities in patients with TBI including those with seizures on ASMs.

Conclusions

Patients with TBI can develop seizures and behavioral disturbance. Gaining an understanding of the side effect profile of ASMs is thus vital in treating this unique subset of patients. The effects of ASMs can be divided into two general categories – cognitive and behavioral. The studies noted throughout this chapter have outlined the positive and negative influences of each ASM on cognition. The ASMs can be separated into medications that result in low, intermediate and high cognitive deficits; they are outlined in Table 13.1. The classification of ASMS as having low, intermediate and high cognitive risks is based on the opinion of the authors' interpretation of the literature. It is a relative estimate and will vary across individuals and other factors such as the underlying cognitive profile of each patient (e.g., baseline abilities and extent of TBI), the other medications they are taking, the dose and blood levels of their ASM(s) and

Table 13.1 Relative potential risks for cognitive side effects from ASMs

Potential cognitive risks	Anti-seizure medications
Low	Brivateracetam, lacosamide, lamotrigine, levetiracetam
Low to intermediate	Gabapentin, elsicarbazepine, perampanel
Intermediate	Carbamazepine, oxcarbazepine, phenytoin, valproate
Intermediate to high	Zonisamide
High	Benzodiazepines, phenobarbital, topiramate

Table 13.2 Relative potential risks for behavioral effects from ASMs

Potential behavioral effects	Anti-seizure medications
Positive	Carbamazepine, gabapentin, lamotrigine, oxcarbazepine, valproate
Neutral	Lacosamide, phenytoin
Negative	Benzodiazepines, brivateracetam, levetiracetam, perampanel, phenobarbital, topiramate, zonisamide

their age. The nature of behavioral effects from ASMs can also be summarized and separated into three separate categories: positive, neutral and negative (outlined in Table 13.2). Careful consideration of the behavioral and cognitive side effects of each anti-seizure medication can allow for the most effective treatment of seizures and improvement in the quality of life in patients with TBI. Further studies to investigate and compare the side effect profiles of ASMs are necessary, and other treatment strategies such as surgery or neurostimulation can be considered in patients who become medically refractory.

References

1. Meador KJ. Cognitive effects of epilepsy and its treatments. In: Wyllie E, Cascino GD, Gidal BE, Goodkin HP, Loddenkemper T, Sirven JI (eds). *Wyllie's Treatment of Epilepsy: Principles & Practice*, 7th Edition. Philadelphia: Lippincott Williams & Wilkins. 2020: 1058–61.

2. Dodrill CB, Troupin AS. Neuropsychological effects of carbamazepine and phenytoin: a reanalysis. *Neurology* 1991;**41**:141–3.

3. Meador KJ, Loring DW, Allen ME, *et al.* Comparative cognitive effects of carbamazepine and phenytoin in healthy adults. *Neurology* 1991;**41**:1537–40.

4. Hessen E, Lossius MI, Reinvang I, *et al.* Influence of major antiepileptic drugs on neuropsychological function: results from a randomized, double- blind, placebo-controlled withdrawal study of seizure-free epilepsy patients on monotherapy. *J Int Neuropsychol Soc* 2007;**13**:393–400.

5. Matagne A, Margineanu DG, Kenda B, Michel P, Klitgaard H. Anti-convulsive and anti-epileptic properties of brivaracetam (UCB 34714),a high-affinity ligand for the synaptic vesicle protein, SV2A. *Br J Pharmacol* 2008;**154**:1662–71.

6. Meador KJ, Gevins A, Leese PT, *et al.* Neurocognitive effects of brivaracetam, levetiracetam, and lorazepam. *Epilepsia* 2011;**52**:264–72.

7. Zahnert F, Krause K, Immisch I, *et al.* Brivaracetam in the treatment of patients with epilepsy-first clinical experiences. *Front Neurol* 2018;**9**:38.

8. Meador KJ, Seliger J, Boyd A, *et al.* Comparative neuropsychological effects of carbamazepine and eslicarbazepine acetate. *Epilepsy Behav* 2019;**94**:151–7.

9. Leach JP, Girvan J, Paul A, *et al.* Gabapentin and cognition: a double-blind, dose-ranging, placebo-controlled study in refractory epilepsy. *J Neurol Neurosurg Psychiatry* 1997;**62**:372–6.

10. Meador KJ, Loring DW, Ray PG, *et al.* Differential cognitive effects of carbamazepine and gabapentin. *Epilepsia* 1999;**40**:1279–85.

11. Salinsky MC, Binder LM, Oken BS, *et al.* Effects of gabapentin and carbamazepine on the EEG and cognition in healthy volunteers. *Epilepsia* 2002;**43**:482–90.

12. Meador KJ, Loring DW, Boyd A, *et al.* Randomized double-blind comparison of

cognitive and EEG effects of lacosamide and carbamazepine. *Epilepsy Behav* 2016;**62**:267–75.

13. Meador KJ, Loring DW, Ray PG, *et al.* Differential cognitive and behavioral effects of carbamazepine and lamotrigine. *Neurology.* 2001;**56**:1177–82.

14. Meador KJ, Loring DW, Vahle VJ, *et al.* Cognitive and behavioral effects of lamotrigine and topiramate in healthy volunteers. *Neurology.* 2005;**64**:2108–14.

15. Aldenkamp AP, Arends J, Bootsma HP, *et al.* Randomized double-blind parallel-group study comparing cognitive effects of a low-dose lamotrigine with valproate and placebo in healthy volunteers. *Epilepsia* 2002; **43**:19–26.

16. Cohen AF, Ashby L, Crowley D, *et al.* Lamotrigine (BW430C), a potential anticonvulsant. Effects on the central nervous system in comparison with phenytoin and diazepam. *Br J Clin Pharmacol* 1985;**20**:619–29.

17. Hamilton MJ, Cohen AF, Yuen AW, *et al.* Carbamazepine and lamotrigine in healthy volunteers: relevance to early tolerance and clinical trial dosage. *Epilepsia* 1993;**34**:166–73.

18. Blum D, Meador KJ, Biton V, *et al.* Cognitive effects of lamotrigine compared with topiramate in patients with epilepsy. *Neurology* 2006;**67**:400–6.

19. Vajda FJ, Dodd S, Horgan D. Lamotrigine in epilepsy, pregnancy and psychiatry: a drug for all seasons? *J Clin Neurosci* 2013;**20**:13–16.

20. Meador KJ, Gevins A, Loring DW, *et al.* Neuropsychological and neurophysiological effects of carbamazepine and levetiracetam. *Neurology* 2007;**69**:2076–84.

21. Labiner DM, Ettinger AB, Fakhoury TA, *et al.* Effects of lamotrigine compared with levetiracetam on anger, hostility, and total mood in patients with partial epilepsy. *Epilepsia* 2009;**50**:434–42.

22. Marino S, Vitaliti G, Marino SD, *et al.* Pyridoxine add-on treatment for the control of behavioral adverse effects induced by levetiracetam in children: A case–control prospective study. *Ann Pharmacother*, 2018;**52**, 645–9.

23. Donati F, Gobbi G, Campistol J, *et al.* The cognitive effects of oxcarbazepine versus carbamazepine or valproate in newly diagnosed children with partial seizures. *Seizure* 2007;**16**:670–9.

24. Aikia M, Kalviainen R, Sivenius J, *et al.* Cognitive effects of oxcarbazepine and phenytoin monotherapy in newly diagnosed epilepsy: one year follow-up. *Epilepsy Res* 1992;**11**:199–203.

25. Salinsky MC, Spencer DC, Oken BS, *et al.* Effects of oxcarbazepine and phenytoin on the EEG and cognition in healthy volunteers. *Epilepsy Behav* 2004;**5**:894–902.

26. Meador KJ, Yang H, Piña-Garza JE, *et al.* Cognitive effects of adjunctive perampanel for partial-onset seizures: A randomized trial. *Epilepsia* 2016;**57**:243–51.

27. Piña-Garza JE, Lagae L, Villanueva V, *et al.* Long-term effects of adjunctive perampanel on cognition in adolescents with partial seizures. *Epilepsy Behav* 2018;**83**:50–8.

28. Aldenkamp AP, Alpherts WC. The effect of the new antiepileptic drug rufinamide on cognitive functions. *Epilepsia* 2006;**47**:1153–9.

29. Dodrill CB, Arnett JL, Sommerville K, *et al.* Cognitive and quality of life effects of differing dosages of tiagabine in epilepsy. *Neurology* 1997;**48**:1025–31.

30. Sharief M, Viteri C, Ben-Menachem E, *et al.* Double-blind, placebo-controlled study of topiramate in patients with refractory partial epilepsy. *Epilepsy Res* 1996;**25**:217–24.

31. Tassinari CA, Michelucci R, Chauvel P, *et al.* Double-blind, placebo-controlled trial of topiramate (600 mg daily) for the treatment of refractory partial epilepsy. *Epilepsia* 1996;**37**:763–86.

32. Ben-Menachim E, Henriksen O, Dam M, Schmidt D. Double-blind, placebo-controlled trial of topiramate as add-on therapy in patients with refractory partial seizures. *Epilepsia* 1996;**37**:539–43.

33. Faught E, Wilder BJ, Ramsay RE, *et al.* Topiramate placebo- controlled dose-ranging trial in refractory partial epilepsy using 200,400, and 600-mg daily dosages. *Neurology* 1996;**46**: 1684–90.

34. Aldenkamp AP, Baker G, Mulder OG, *et al.* A multicenter, randomized clinical study to evaluate the effect on cognitive function of topiramate compared with valproate as add-on therapy to carbamazepine in patients with partial-onset seizures. *Epilepsia* 2000;**41**:1167–78.

35. Meador KJ, Loring DW, Hulihan JF, *et al.* Differential cognitive and behavioral effects of topiramate and valproate. *Neurology* 2003;**60**:1483–8.

36. Salinsky MC, Storzbach D, Spencer DC, *et al.* Effects of topiramate and gabapentin on cognitive abilities in healthy volunteers. *Neurology* 2005;**64**:792–8.

37. Loring DW, Williamson DJ, Meador KJ, *et al.* Topiramate dose effects on cognition: a randomized double-blind study. *Neurology* 2011;**76**: 131–7.

38. Ferrie CD, Robinson RO, Panayiotopoulos CP. Psychotic and severe behavioural reactions with vigabatrin: a review. *Acta Neurol Scand* 1996;**93**:1–8.

39. Dodrill CB, Arnett JL, Sommerville KW, *et al.* Effects of differing dosages of vigabatrin (Sabril) on cognitive abilities and quality of life in epilepsy. *Epilepsia* 1995;**36**:164–73.

40. Grunewald RA, Thompson PJ, Corcoran R, *et al.* Effects of vigabatrin on partial seizures and cognitive function. *J Neurol Neurosurg Psychiatr* 1994;**57**:1057–63.

41. Berent S, Sackellares JC, Giordani B, *et al.* Zonisamide (CI-912) and cognition: results from preliminary study. *Epilepsia.* 1987;**28**:61–67. 2008;**12**:102–108.

42. Park SP, Hwang YH, Lee HW, et al. Long-term cognitive and mood effects of zonisamide monotherapy in epilepsy patients. *Epilepsy & Behavior* 2008;**12**:102–8.

43. Wiebe S, Blume W, Girvin J, Eliasziw M. A randomized, controlled trial of surgery for temporal-lobe epilepsy. *N Engl J Med* 2001;**345**:311–18

44. Dulay, M. Busch, R. Prediction of neuropsychological outcome after resection of temporal and extratemporal seizure foci. *Neurosurg Focus* 2012;**32**:E4.

45. Chan A, Rolston J, Rao, V. and Chang E. Effect of neurostimulation on cognition and mood in refractory epilepsy. *Epilepsia Open*, 2018, **3**:18–29.

46. Hoppe C, Helmstaedter C, Scherrmann J, *et al.* No evidence for cognitive side effects after 6 months of vagus nerve stimulation in epilepsy patients. *Epilepsy Behav* 2001;**2**:351–6.

47. Tröster AI, Meador KJ, Irwin CP, *et al.* Memory and mood outcomes after anterior thalamic stimulation for refractory partial epilepsy. *Seizure* 2017;**45**:133–41.

48. Loring DW, Kapur R, Meador KJ, *et al.* Differential neuropsychological outcomes following targeted responsive neurostimulation for partial-onset epilepsy. *Epilepsia* 2015; **56**:1836–44.

49. Adams J, Alipio-Jocson V, Inoyama K, *et al.* Methylphenidate, cognition, and epilepsy: A double-blind, placebo-controlled, single-dose study. *Neurology* 2017;**88**:470–6.

50. Adams J, Alipio-Jocson V, Inoyama K, *et al.* Methylphenidate, cognition, and epilepsy: A 1-month open-label trial. *Epilepsia* 2017;**58**:2124–32.

51. Liu X, Carney PR, Bussing R, Segal R, Cottler LB, Winterstein AG. Stimulants do not increase the risk of seizure-related hospitalizations in children with epilepsy. *J Child Adolesc Psychopharmacol* 2018;**28**:111–16.

52. Wiggs KK, Chang Z, Quinn PD, *et al.* Attention-deficit/hyperactivity disorder medication and seizures. *Neurology* 2018;**90**:e1104–10.

Post-traumatic Epilepsy in Low Income Countries

Jeevagan Vijayabala

History

Post-traumatic epilepsy (PTE) was recognized in ancient India several thousand years ago. Epilepsy was mentioned using the terms *Apasmara* or *Apasmrti* in many Ayurvedic texts dating to 2500 BC and earlier.[1] There have been three factors commonly implicated for the etiology of *Apasmara*: endogenous factors (genetic, congenital and enzymatic disturbances); exogenous factors (intake of unwholesome and unhygienic foods, worms and other environmental factors including trauma); and psychological factors (excessive worry, anger and anxiety).[2] According to ancient literature the aggravated *vata dosa* (one of the life-forces which govern flow and motion in the body) due to brain trauma spreads throughout the body through nerves, leading to manifestation of post-traumatic seizures in the form of shaking limbs (*akshepaka*) or episodes of brief unconsciousness without shaking (*apatantraka*).[2] The ancient literature also concludes that PTE can only be controlled with medications and can sometimes be incurable and will remain uncontrolled.

Burden

Traumatic brain injury (TBI) is the one of the leading cause of death especially in younger people in many developing countries.[3] Health systems in low and middle income countries are not prepared well to tackle the post-traumatic consequences including PTE. The data on epidemiology, financial costs and the social impact of PTE is sparse.[4] Increased incidence of road traffic accidents, combined with poor healthcare services, as well as lack of knowledge of the causes and consequences are underlying causes for the disproportionately high burden of PTE in those countries.[5]

Epidemiology

Epidemiological data on incidence, prevalence and mortality of PTE is particularly important for optimal health care delivery and prevention of this condition. Poverty and poor national health resources are major reasons for the inadequate number of neuro-epidemiological studies in the developing world where more than half of the world's population resides. Inaccuracy of death certification is another reason for unreliability of the mortality data for PTE in these areas. Lack of a universal definition on PTE also contributes to lack of epidemiological data. Starting anti-epileptic drugs (AEDs) as prophylaxis following TBI and prescribing AEDs for acute symptomatic seizures may lead to methodological flaws. In contrast to developed countries, lack of centralized reporting systems or national disease registries together with inadequate population-based studies makes obtaining reliable statistics on PTE a daunting task.

Epidemiology of TBI

The leading causes for TBI in most of the developing world are road traffic accidents, assaults and accidental falls.[6] Almost two-thirds of TBI cases occur due to traffic accidents, and the other onethird of cases are mainly due to violence/assault and accidental falls.

Road Traffic Accidents

Road traffic injury is a leading cause of death and disability among adolescents and young adults in many developing countries. It is estimated more than 85% of all deaths due to motor vehicle crashes occur in developing countries.[7] There are multiple reasons for dramatic increase in traffic-related case fatalities. The recent growth in numbers of motor vehicles without infrastructure development is a major cause for rising fatalities from traffic-related injuries in poor countries. Extensive use of public transport and prevalence of poor quality vehicles which often carry more people than their authorized capacity are two main factors contributing to comparatively higher proportion of death toll in these countries.[8] There are number of other factors associated with increased incidence of motor vehicle crashes, such as poor practice of road safety measures, high speed driving, low level of vehicle ownership and inadequate public health infrastructure.[9, 10] The highest burden of morbidity and mortality is borne disproportionately by poor people, as pedestrians, passengers of public transport and cyclists are more vulnerable. It is estimated that urban pedestrians account for around two-third of deaths.[11, 12]

Violence

Many developing countries suffer or have suffered large-scale war and violence. Both civilians and security personnel residing near war zones are more prone to develop TBI as well as other life-threatening injuries.[13] Increased use of improvised explosive devices results in high number of blast injuries and closed head injuries.[14] TBI often goes unnoticed when it occurs without any signs of external injuries.

Higher prevalence of alcohol consumption due to increasing availability without proper regulation contributes to increased rate of violence (with or without weapons) in those countries.[15] In some countries around quarter of TBI occurred under influence of alcohol. It is estimated that morbidity and disability due to TBI are almost twice the rate than in those who were not under the influence of alcohol.[16]

Falls

Around 424,000 fall-related fatalities occur globally each year.[17] It is estimated that more than 80% of those fatalities occur in developing countries.[18] Around 20% to 30% of fallers sustain TBI.[19] People at the extremities of age are more vulnerable to fall-related injuries. It is imperative to have better understanding of unique contributors of falls in the elderly and in children.

The elderly population continues to rise in many developing countries. Around two-thirds of the hospitalizations due to injuries in elders are due to falls.[20] Elders in these countries are more vulnerable to falls and fall-related injuries due to malnutrition, hazards at home, environmental risk factors, lack of accessible transportation and inadequate health services.[21] The cost of fall-related injuries and their burden on health care systems are disproportionately high in low income countries.

Most fall-related injuries in pediatric population occur while playing either at home or school. Children are often unattended without adequate safety measures. Lack of knowledge and appreciation by parents further increases the chances for falls.[22] A study from China revealed that for every pediatric death from a fall, there were four children with a permanent disability and 37 requiring hospitalization.[23]

Occupational health hazards are the main contributing factors to falls in the middle-age population.[24] Worker safety remains an important health problem in many low and middle income countries. Financial constrains lead to unsafe work practices. Falls from height at construction sites are a common cause of TBI, leading to higher mortality and morbidity.[25]

Epidemiology of Post-traumatic Epilepsy

As post-traumatic epilepsy (PTE) is the one of the common complications of TBI, rising rate of TBI has resulted in increased incidence of PTE in many developing countries. However, studies on incidence of PTE in developing countries are very rare. Available small-scale studies reported incidence of PTE ranging from 2.5% to 5%.

In a cohort of 520 TBI patients in India, overall 11.4% developed post-traumatic seizure (PTS). Most of them (8.9% of the whole cohort) developed seizures within a week of TBI.[26] Independent risk factors for PTS were severity of TBI at presentation, associated medical comorbidities and fall from height. During the median follow-up of 386 days, 32.2% of patients with PTS developed recurrence seizures. The recurrence was higher in patients with late-onset seizures, while multiple early seizures were not associated with long-term recurrence.

In a Chinese cohort of 2,826 TBI patients, the incidence of PTE was 5% during the first 3 years after the trauma.[27] In addition to the severity of TBI, other factors associated with increased incidence of PTE were older age, abnormal neuroimaging and surgical interventions. In contrast to the Indian study, around 66.7% of the victims with acute and early seizures developed PTE.

In another multicenter Chinese study, the overall incidence of PTS was 9.8% among 3,093 patients during the 2-year follow up[28]; 35.1% developed seizures while they were in hospital. More than half (59.9%) of them were diagnosed as having PTS at 6 months. Only 21.9% developed PTS after 1 year. Severity of TBI, frontal-temporal lobar contusion and linear fracture are risk factors for PTS.

A survey of 163 Iranian war veterans with intractable epilepsy revealed that the PTS occurred earlier in patients with penetrating trauma (78% developed within 1 year) in comparison with blunt trauma cases (only 38% had seizure within 1 year).[29] In addition, seizure frequency and duration of unconsciousness were higher in veterans who sustained penetrating trauma.

As there are differences in sample size, study setting, mechanisms and severity of the injury, it is not possible to draw any reliable conclusion from the studies described here.

Mechanisms of PTE

The pathophysiology of PTE is not simple and involves both primary and secondary brain injury mechanisms. It may differ between penetrating injuries and closed head injuries.

The Vietnam Head Injury study confirm the association between penetrating TBI and PTS. Out of the 421 veterans who suffered TBI, 53% developed PTE.[30] The majority of cases developed within a year of TBI and almost half of them were still experiencing seizures 15 years after their TBI. Focal neurological signs, large lesions and presence of hematoma and retained metal fragments were associated with increased risk of developing PTE. Only lesions in some parts of brain, such as left temporal gray matter/hippocampus, right vertex gray matter, significantly predicted seizure occurrence.

An animal model of penetrating TBI in rats closely resembles the many aspects of war-time TBI.[31] A computer operated hydraulic pressure generator was used to simulate the two aspects of a high-energy bullet injury to brain: a permanent injury tract created by the path of the bullet and the large temporary cavity generated by energy dissipation of the penetrating bullet. Up to 70% of rats developed one or more seizures 72 hours after injury, and the frequency and duration of epileptic events correlated with the severity of the injury. Pathological examination revealed a penumbral zone of injury surrounding the core zone of injury susceptible to secondary injury.

The Fluid Percussion Injury model (FPI) mimics the pathophysiology of closed head injury by reproducing both destructive processes and regenerative inflammatory processes.[32] Conventionally, injury is induced by rapid fluid injection through a craniotomy combined with a hammer swung on a pendulum. A group of researchers from China recently evaluated an advanced device for FPI in rats.[33] The device was software controlled and delivered more reliable fluid percussion pulses. FPI-induced electrographic as well as clinical seizures.

Management of PTE

Access to appropriate treatment for PTE is poor in developing countries. PTE in many developing countries is often managed by general physicians due to lack of specialist neurologists or epileptologists. Such specialists are often concentrated in urban areas giving rise to a large treatment gap in rural areas. In addition to the lack of specialists, high costs of treatment, increased distance to health care facilities, inadequate knowledge about PTE and stigmatization also contribute to unacceptably high treatment gap.

The diagnosis of PTE is made on clinical grounds. Diagnostic tests such as electroencephalography (EEG), computed tomography (CT) scan and magnetic resonance imaging (MRI) scan may assist in the assessment of patients with PTE.[34] In the acute setting, a CT scan is effective in the assessment of moderate to severe TBI, but MRI is the imaging modality of choice for mild TBI and for patients with PTE. Even though MRI is available in many developing countries, its accessibility is limited to private health care facilities in larger cities. Long-term video EEG monitoring is not available in many low income countries. Furthermore, interpretation of EEG can be challenging in the absence of adequate number of specialists.

The American Academy of Neurology recommends prophylactic treatment with phenytoin for first 7 days for patients with severe TBI (typically with prolonged loss of consciousness or amnesia, intracranial hematoma or brain contusion on CT scan and/or depressed skull fracture).[35] Although phenytoin has been shown to decrease the incidence of early PTS, this treatment does not protect against late PTS or PTE.[36] In a retrospective analysis in China, effectiveness of sodium valproate for the prevention of early PTS was evaluated.[37] Out of 87 severe TBI patients, 6 patients in the control group developed early PTS whereas no patient from the sodium valproate cohort developed early seizures. The authors concluded that sodium valproate was effective in decreasing the risk of early seizures in severe TBI. However, the difference was not statistically significant. Furthermore, a previous randomized trial in Washington revealed tend toward a higher mortality rate among TBI patients treated with sodium valproate.[38]

A small scale single blinded randomized trial showed that use of levetiracetam may be associated with better cognitive outcome in comparison with phenytoin.[39] Many second generation antiepileptic drugs including levetiracetam are not available in many resource-limited countries. Despite having a better safety profile, many patients in poor countries do not receive newer antiepileptic medications suitable for their needs and comorbidities.[40]

Summary and Conclusion

Increased incidence of TBI due to rising rate of road traffic injuries, violence and falls has resulted in comparatively higher prevalence of PTE in developing world. However, the absence of reliable epidemiological data precludes statistical comparisons. At the same time, the majority of patients with epilepsy do not receive appropriate medical treatment due to poverty and poor health infrastructure. Understanding the barriers to epilepsy care delivery is paramount to improve the quality of care of the patients with PTE. More weight also should be given to primary prevention tactics tailored for developing nations to curtail the incidence of TBI and resultant PTE.

References

1. Tandon PN. Ayurveda and epilepsy. In: Tandon PN, ed. *Epilepsy in India: Report based on a multicentric study on epidemiology of epilepsy carried out as a PL 480 funded project of the Indian Council of Medical Research*, New Delhi, India, 1989:176–80.

2. Bhatt HA, Gogtay NJ, Dalvi SS, Kshirsagar NA. Epilepsy. In: Mishra LC, ed: *Scientific Basis for Ayurvedic therapies*. Washington DC: CRC Press, 2003:427–37

3. Puvanachandra P, Hyder AA. The burden of traumatic brain injury in Asia: A call for research. *Pak J Neurol Sci* 2009;4(1):27–32

4. GBD 2016 Neurology Collaborators Global, regional, and national burden of traumatic brain injury and spinal cord injury, 1990–2016: a systematic analysis for the Global Burden of Disease Study 2016. *Lancet Neurol* 2019;18:56–87.

5. El-Gindi S, Mahdy M, Abdel Azeem A. Traumatic brain injury in developing countries. Road war in Africa. *Rev Esp Neuropsicol* 2001;3:3–11.

6. Murray CJ, López AD. *The Global burden of disease: a comprehensive assessment of mortality and disability from diseases, injuries, and risk factors in 1990 and projected in 2020 Boston*: Harvard School of Public Health: Harvard University Press, 1996.

7. Krug EG (ed). Injury: a leading cause of the global burden of disease. World Health Organization. 1999. https://apps.who.int/iris/handle/10665/66160.

8. Nantulya VM, Muli-Musiime F. Kenya. Uncovering the social determinants of road traffic accidents. In: Evans T, Whitehead M, Diderichsen F, Bhuiya A, Wirth M, eds. *Challenging Inequities: from Ethics to Action*. Oxford: Oxford University Press, 2001.

9. Odero W, Garner P, Zwi A. Road traffic injuries in developing countries: a comprehensive review of epidemiological studies. *Trop Med Int Health* 1997;2:445–60.

10. Kapila S, Manundu M, Lamba D. The "matatu" mode of public transport in metropolitan Nairobi. Nairobi: Mazingira Institute Report, 1982.

11. Mock CN, NII-Amon-Kotei D, Maier RV. Low utilization of formal medical services by injured persons in a developing nation: health service data underestimate the importance of trauma. *J Trauma* 1997;42:504–13.

12. Mohan D, Tiwari G. Traffic safety in low-income countries: issues and concerns

regarding technology transfer from high-income countries. In: *Reflections of the Transfer of Traffic Safety Knowledge to Motorizing Nations*. Melbourne: Global Safety Trust, 1998:27–56.

13. Stewart F, Fitzgerald V, eds. *War and Underdevelopment: the Economic and Social Consequences of Conflict*. Oxford: Oxford University Press, 2001.

14. Lindquist LK, Love HC, Elbogen EB. Traumatic brain injury in Iraq and Afghanistan veterans: New results from a national random sample Study. *J Neuropsychiatry Clin Neurosci*. 2017;29:254–9.

15. Girish N, Kavita R, Gururaj G, Benegal V. Alcohol use and implications for public health: patterns of use in four communities. *Indian J Community Med* 2010;35:238–44.

16. Gururaj G. Epidemiology of traumatic brain injuries: Indian scenario. *Neurol Res*. 2002;24(1):24–8.

17. Peden M, McGee K, Sharma G. *The Injury Chart Book: A Graphical Overview of the Global Burden of Injuries*. Geneva: World Health Organization;2002.

18. Mathers C, Boerma T, Ma Fat D. *The Global Burden of Disease* 2004 update. Geneva: World Health Organization;2008.

19. Gupta S, Gupta SK, Devkota S, *et al*. Fall Injuries in Nepal: A countrywide population-based survey. *Ann Glob Health*. 2015;81:487–94.

20. Kalula SZ, Scott V, Dowd A, Brodrick K. Falls and fall prevention programmes in developing countries: environmental scan for the adaptation of the Canadian Falls prevention curriculum for developing countries. *J Safety Res* 2011;42:461–72.

21. Kalula SZ. *A WHO Global Report on Falls among Older Persons: Prevention of Falls in Older Persons: Africa Case Study*. World Health Organization. 2008.

22. Bhatti JA, Farooq U, Majeed M, et al. Fall-related injuries in a low-income setting: Results from a pilot injury surveillance system in Rawalpindi, Pakistan. *J Epidemiol Glob Health* 2015;5:283–90.

23. World Health Organization. Children and Falls. Available at: www.who.int/violence_injury_prevention/child/injury/world_report/Falls_english.pdf. Accessed January 3, 2020.

24. Grivna M, Eid HO, Abu-Zidan FM. Epidemiology, morbidity and mortality from fall-related injuries in the United Arab Emirates. *Scand J Trauma Resusc Emerg Med* 2014;22:51.

25. Nadhim EA, Hon C, Xia B, Stewart I, Fang D. Falls from height in the construction industry: A critical review of the scientific literature. *Int J Environ Res Public Health* 2016;13(7):638.

26. Thapa A, Chandra SP, Sinha S, Sreenivas V, Sharma BS, Tripathi M. Post-traumatic seizures-A prospective study from a tertiary level trauma center in a developing country. *Seizure* 2010;19(4):211–6.

27. Zhao Y, Wu H, Wang X, Li J, Zhang S. Clinical epidemiology of posttraumatic epilepsy in a group of Chinese patients. *Seizure* 2012;21(5):322–6.

28. Wang H, Xin T, Sun X, *et al*. Post-traumatic seizures–a prospective, multicenter, large case study after head injury in China. *Epilepsy Res* 2013;107(3):272–8.

29. Kazemi H, Hashemi-Fesharaki S, Razaghi S, *et al*. Intractable epilepsy and craniocerebral trauma: analysis of 163 patients with blunt and penetrating head injuries sustained in war. *Injury* 2012;43:2132–5.

30. Salazar, JB, Vance SC, *et al*. Epilepsy after penetrating head injury. Clinical correlates: a report of the Vietnam head injury study. *Neurology*1985;35:1406–14.

31. Williams AJ, Hartings JA, Lu XC, Rolli ML, Dave JR, Tortella FC. Characterization of a new rat model of penetrating ballistic brain injury. *J Neurotrauma* 2005;22:313–31.

32. Bao YH, Bramlett HM, Atkins CM, et al. Post-traumatic seizures exacerbate histopathological damage after

fluid-percussion brain injury. *J Neurotrauma* 2011;28:35–42.

33. Ouyang W, Wu W, Fan Z, Wang J, Pan H, Yang W. Modified device for fluid percussion injury in rodents. *J Neurosci Res* 2018;96:1412–29.

34. Piccenna L, Shears G, O'Brien TJ. Management of post-traumatic epilepsy: An evidence review over the last 5 years and future directions. *Epilepsia Open* 2017;2(2):123–44.

35. Chang BS, Lowenstein DH. Quality Standards Subcommittee of the American Academy of Neurology. Practice parameter: antiepileptic drug prophylaxis in severe traumatic brain injury: report of the Quality Standards Subcommittee of the American Academy of Neurology. *Neurology* 2003;60:10.

36. Schierhout G, Roberts I. Anti-epileptic drugs for preventing seizures following acute traumatic brain injury. *Cochrane Database Syst Rev* 2001;CD000173.

37. Ma CY, Xue YJ, Li M, Zhang Y, Li GZ. Sodium valproate for prevention of early posttraumatic seizures. *Chin J Traumatol* 2010;13:293–6.

38. Temkin NR1, Dikmen SS, Anderson GD, et al. Valproate therapy for prevention of posttraumatic seizures: a randomized trial. *J Neurosurg* 1999;91:593–600.

39. Szaflarski JP, Sangha KS, Lindsell CJ, Shutter LA. Prospective, randomized, single-blinded comparative trial of intravenous levetiracetam versus phenytoin for seizure prophylaxis. *Neurocrit Care* 2010;12: 165–72.

40. Trinka E, Kwan P, Lee B, Dash A. Epilepsy in Asia: Disease burden, management barriers, and challenges. *Epilepsia*. 2019;60 Suppl 1:7–21.

Index